WEIGHT LOSS MEDICAL COOKBOOK

Mediterranean Gourmet Recipes with Medical & Nutritional Guidance from Dr. Jaime Durand

Jaime Durand, M.D.
&
Carmen Rosa Arias Schreiber

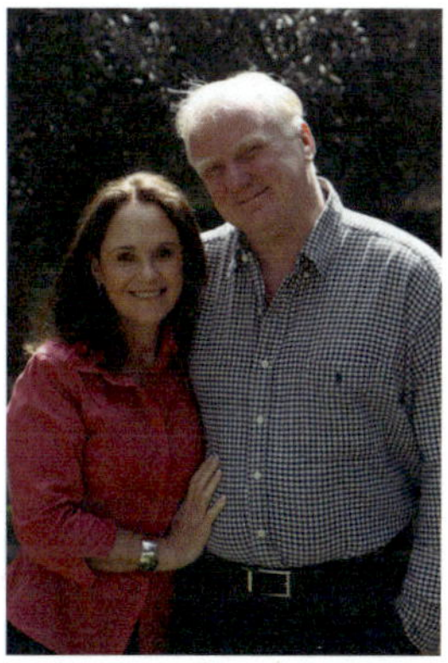

Concept, Research and Direction
Dr. Jaime Durand and Carmen Rosa Arias Schreiber

General Coordination
Carmen Rosa Arias Schreiber

Medical-Dietician Consulting
Dr. Jaime Durand and Dr. Cecilia Kineche

Culinary and Food Elaboration Advice
Carmen Rosa Arias Schreiber and Chef Marcelo Portuondo

Editing and Design
Liliana Arias Schreiber de Cardenas

Production
Jaime Durand MD PA

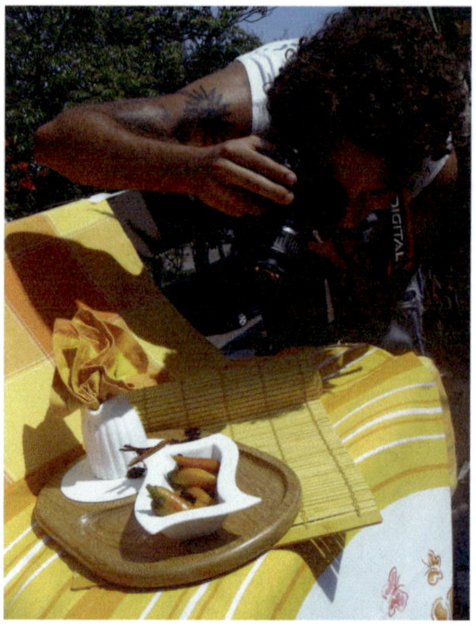

Photography
Mauricio Gil

ISBN 0-9844149-0-8
www.weightlossmedicalcookbook.com

JAIME DURAND, MD

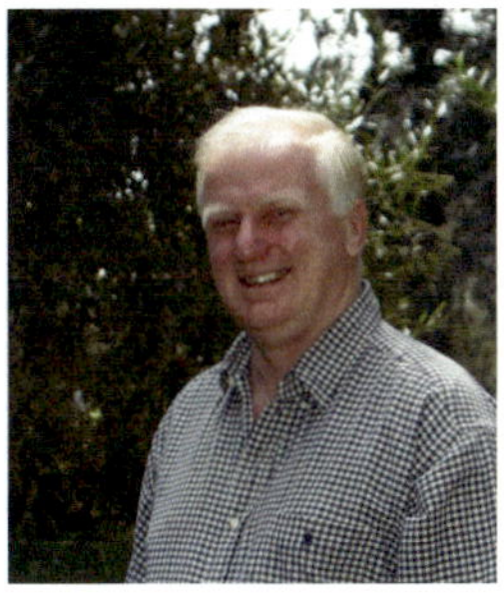

Jaime Durand, MD, is a Board Certified physician specializing in Internal Medicine (1986), Rheumatology (1988) and Geriatric Medicine (1992). He has over 30 years of experience practicing clinical medicine, and currently works with patients at the Rheumatic & Connective Tissue Disease Clinic of Arlington in Texas. He is affiliated with the Medical Center of Arlington and Plaza Hospital in Fort Worth, Texas.

He has extensive experience treating arthritis, pain, injury and allied conditions, and offers complete diagnostic and treatment expertise to patients suffering from collagen-vascular and auto-immune diseases, as well as metabolic and genetic conditions leading to arthritis, bone diseases and systemic or local injury to the body.

Dr. Durand began with a scientific research-oriented career in immunology, which led to the development of a strong clinical practice specializing in geriatric and rheumatological patients. He has strong connections to medical institutions in the United States as well as abroad. He is a member (fellow) of the *American College of Rheumatology, American Geriatric Society*, *American Association of Physicians and Surgeons*, *Colegio Médico del Perú*, *Sociedad Peruana de Medicina Interna* and *Sociedad Peruana de Geriatría.* He speaks Spanish fluently, and is committed to the development of a healthy Hispanic American community in Texas. He is an advocate of a free market medical environment for the medical profession, and has a strong political vocation towards the development of a stronger democratic system for America.

Dr. Durand was born in Lima, Peru, and graduated from Cayetano Heredia University, Lima, Peru, in 1981.

Internship and Residency:
- Henry Ford Hospital (July 1982 – June 1984)
- Sinai Hospital of Detroit (July 1984 – June 1986) in Detroit, Michigan

He completed his Rheumatology Fellowship in the Rheumatology Department at University of Texas Southwestern Medical School Health Science Center in Dallas (June 1988), and his Geriatric Fellowship was completed at Loyola University-Hines VA in Chicago, Illinois.

Dr. Durand is the senior Medical Director of the Residencia Médica El Olivar, Rheumatological and Geriatric Clinical Research Center in Lima, Peru.

He has provided Geriatric Service for the Department of Veterans Affairs at John F Kennedy VA Hospital at Memphis (December, 1989) and at Edward Hines Jr. VA Hospital in Hines, Illinois (June 1991).

Carmen Rosa Arias Schreiber was born in Lima, Peru, and currently resides in the United States. A landscaper for more than 15 years in her country of origin, her interest in cooking and health led to the creation and testing of the recipes included here.

She adapted the Mediterranean Diet to America's fast-paced culture in order to facilitate weight loss and vibrant health for patients of Dr. Durand. This book contains a practical application of the highly acclaimed diet, rich with photos and easy to understand techniques for both the novice and skilled cook.

TABLE OF CONTENTS

PROLOGUE

This book is a love story about food …

The thought of having to move from Lima, Peru, to the United States at my age made me very weary. Leaving my daughters, parents, siblings and friends gave me a feeling of extreme loneliness. Or even worse, I believed that adaptation, if it occurred, would be very slow and hard.

In retrospect, I think my greatest advantage was a clear mind-set for living a new life. With my past behind and a promising future at hand I arrived at the city of Arlington, Texas, several years ago.

What did this future I had postponed so many times offered me? Actually, much more than what I had imagined. I soon realized that sharing my life with my fiancé happened to be very pleasant, and that adapting to my new life was an amusing situation, rich with new experiences.

There was peace in my soul and I was calm enough to understand that my loved ones were doing well. And should they need me, thanks to the magic of modern telecommunication, at any time doubts were solved, decisions were taken and, in spite of our distance, our lives kept rolling in their usual path.

Although my days were good, there were moments of intense loneliness and sadness. I remember that in order to feel better and get away from the negative feelings (characteristic of those who live in foreign lands) I found a unique pleasure in buying and devouring the most provocative processed foods that crammed the supermarkets in this country.

All this was new to me. Although I had come to the United States for short stays on several occasions, I was now living there and the need to explore the numerous foods in attractive colorful boxes became enthralling.

Even the organic foods supermarket in the city became my sanctuary. Not 2 or 3 days would go by and there I was again finding out what was new on the shelves. The cheese section, the chocolates and cookies from all corners of the world, became my obsession. At any occasion, eating junk food, even if not my favorite, gave me no remorse at all.

A few months went by, and my hankering for fast food began to take its toll. Not only was I not feeling well, but I started gaining weight. The clothes that I had brought from Lima were not fitting me any longer and I had to buy clothes 1 or 2 sizes larger than usual. A feeling of anger and frustration started to affect me and I realized all I could do to help myself was return to the eating habits I was raised with.

The Peruvian culture and lifestyle is different particularly in the way we eat. Our region is privileged and generous when it comes to food. Eating seafood, vegetables and fresh fruit is part of our millennial heritage.

Although I was well aware of what I should do, I did not know how to start to reduce my portion sizes and change my already acquired taste for fast food. I began by buying and eating vegetables, fruit, chicken and fish, but I kept on buying and cooking the other foods for my fiancé. In other words, I was making two kinds of meals at the same time, which made reaching my goal far more difficult.

After trying to lose weight for some weeks and failing miserably, I felt something was afoul. If I wanted to succeed I had to involve my partner and eliminate any forbidden food from the fridge and the pantry.

I also had to create a weekly menu that included 3 meals a day, with the list of all the food ingredients we were going to consume. Once a week I had to spend several hours to buy only the foods on the list and store them in a way that would make my daily kitchen work easier.

The first two weeks were the hardest because we had to adjust to smaller portions, and above all, to different flavors. Going to bed early and not having a supply of tempting foods gave us good results, as that kept us away from sleepwalking to the kitchen.

I was excited with the impact of preparing meals swiftly, knowing that a little organization had simplified my life; furthermore, I was beginning to recover my health and reduce my weight.

We discovered diet gelatin was a good ally for hunger attacks and rice cakes were also very helpful. Chicken or vegetable soups were healthy options and quenched our appetite before dining.

Our frequent restaurant incursions, particularly during the first two weeks, were replaced by a delicious salmon fillet, or a tasty homemade chicken breast. The most precious to me was the feeling of complicity and mutual support that arose from this weight loss effort, as it strengthened our relationship even further.

Three weeks had scarcely gone by when we started to notice the changes. We gradually began to lose weight and improve our eating habits. We walked in the evenings and allowed ourselves to eat in some restaurants, although our portions and the type of food we chose had changed. We were adjusting our meals to our new diet.

Over time, these habits became our lifestyle and served as a model for my partner's patients, who were surprised by his continued weight loss. We had unconsciously inspired our eating habits in the Mediterranean diet which, with a few modifications, was producing excellent results.

This first book is born based on the practice of our own experience, on scientific knowledge and research, and from what we know and understand as healthy foods. In this book you will find medical information and simple gourmet recipes, all of them inspired by the healthy Mediterranean diet.

I hope you enjoy eating the Mediterranean diet we present and discover the pleasant aftertaste of natural food, the simplicity of its dishes, the delicious flavors, lovely colors, soft textures and tempting aromas. With some imagination and a small dose of art, eating healthy food can become an experience which is pleasant to your senses and beneficial to your health.

Carmen Rosa Arias-Schreiber

INTRODUCTION

History of the Mediterranean Diet

The Mediterranean diet became popular after World War II. In those years it was already known that the population of Crete had the lowest cardiovascular disease mortality rate.

The seven countries

Based on this background, an epidemiological study entitled *"The Seven Countries Study"* was carried out in the 1960's to investigate the dietary habits of the United States, Japan, Finland, Holland, the former Yugoslavia, Italy and Greece. There were only three countries from the Mediterranean Sea region. The research focused on diet and did not consider the genetic or lifestyle differences of the different populations.

The results of the study demonstrated a clear relationship between diet and the health characteristics of those populations. What was found was that the habitants of Greece, especially those from Crete and southern Italy had the lowest mortality rate from cardiovascular disease and the longest life expectancy. Finland appeared at the opposite end of the spectrum. The United States ranked in an intermediate position, despite being a country that had better living conditions and superior medical services.

Dietary pattern

The healthy characteristics of the Greek diet, especially attributed to the foods of the Cretans and southern Italians, came to be known in the early sixties as the Mediterranean Diet, so named by Doctor Ancel Keys, the scientist who headed the above mentioned study and specialized in epidemiology.

Common characteristics

Later studies showed that there is not just one Mediterranean Diet because the products vary considerably from one country to another. For example, each country consumes different amounts of olive oil. However, it can be stated that the diet of the European countries located on the Mediterranean (Portugal, Spain, southern France, Italy, Greece, etc.) have some common characteristics:

1. Low in saturated fats
2. High in mono-unsaturated fats
3. Balanced in poly-unsaturated acids (Omega-6 and Omega-3)
4. Low in animal protein
5. Rich in anti-oxidants

6. Rich in fibers
7. Low in sugar, especially in simple sugars

These populations consume a comparatively high amount of fish and white meat, but little red meat. They consume cereals, legumes, fruit, and vegetables and drink wine in moderation with meals.

It should be pointed out that the best nourished inhabitants of Mediterranean countries are the Cretans, who obtain alpha-linolenic acid by eating wild plants, snails, nuts, fruits (figs) and eggs. They obtain eicosapentaenoic acid (EPA) and docosahexaenoic acid (DHA) mainly from fish, as well as from bird eggs fed with algae and sea snails.

Mediterranean diet adaptation for weight loss and health improvement

In weight loss programs when comparing several hypo-caloric diets, it was surprising to find that the Mediterranean diet, despite its higher fat content ("good fats" from fish, nuts and vegetables) and low amount of carbohydrates, was more effective for weight loss than "traditional" diets. These traditional diets offered a similar total number of calories and contained fewer fats but these fats were classified as *"bad fats" because they are of animal origin* and the diet also included a comparatively larger amount of carbohydrates.

Results were correlated in research patients with the type of cholesterol and triglycerides measured in their blood. Those who consumed the hypo-caloric Mediterranean diet had a higher proportion of good fats in their blood, HLD or "good cholesterol", than bad fats in blood, LDL or "bad cholesterol".

The hypo-caloric Mediterranean diet with higher content of good fats (mono and poly-unsaturated fats) from fish, nuts and vegetables, produced a much more favorable fasting metabolism than the traditional hypo-caloric diet. This was due to the lower body-oxidation that appeared in these patients compared with the body-oxidation of those who were consuming the traditional hypo-caloric diet, high in sugars and low in bad fats (saturated fats from animal origin).

Despite the higher consumption of good fats, experimental studies in the United States using these two diets have reported a short-term, greater weight loss in patients who consumed the hypo-caloric Mediterranean diet versus those who consumed the traditional low-calorie diet.

However, the same did not happen when the study was extended. Patients who were consuming the hypo-caloric Mediterranean diet gained weight again, while those who were consuming the traditional hypo-caloric diet (low fat) were able to maintain their weight loss.

Because the patients who had begun to reduce their weight by following the hypo-caloric Mediterranean diet did not progressively reduce their portions sizes as they were losing weight, they ended up ingesting more calories than required for their reduced body size.

Consequently, long-term weight loss using the hypo-caloric Mediterranean diet ceased to be effective compared to the other diets. Therefore, the hypo-caloric Mediterranean diet results were considered "invalidated" because it ceased to be a truly hypo-caloric diet for a patient who had already reduced his weight. In this study the traditional hypo-caloric diet maintained weight loss better when used over a longer period of time and resulted in greater weight loss.

It is now understood that patients who are losing weight with the hypo-caloric Mediterranean diet **need to gradually reduce the number of calories consumed** by progressively reducing portion sizes. This diet, still rich in good fats, will maintain its effectiveness.

The dietary therapist who recommends the hypo-caloric Mediterranean diet adapted for weight loss needs to monitor the patient for a longer period of time than generally thought important. This regular monitoring and follow up allows the therapist to gradually reduce food portions, which should correspond to the smaller requirement of calories needed by the decreased mass of the thinner person.

Obesity: a disease of our times

Obesity usually develops in individuals due to a gradual imbalance in their lifestyles and/or to complex changes in biological, emotional, familial, economic and socio-political factors.

Obesity is a growing problem and a modern concern. The eating habits, diet composition, portion sizes, restaurant fare, fast food access and the fact that families seldom sit down to a home cooked meal are all components of the problem.

The shift from farming, manufacturing and other highly physical work to a much more sedentary style of the United States and other developed countries combined with the ease of transportation and the advent of processed and packaged foods have all contributed to the development of obesity and a decreased capacity of the body to use oxygen.

In some first world countries, morbid obesity (that which causes death) has reached epidemic proportions. This phenomenon is particularly noticeable in the United States where the prevalence of overweight, even in children and adolescent populations, has doubled in the last twenty years and tripled in the last forty.

Many of the reasons that hide behind the increase of weight gain and obesity are not easy to determine. What we do know is that the physiological consequences of overweight and obesity affect the individual's life quality, causing problems in the circulatory, respiratory and locomotive systems and even contributing to the apparition of some degenerative diseases such as cancer.

These diseases not only cause premature death to the patient, but create chronic conditions leaving the patient prematurely disabled and with seriously compromised health. This scenario generally creates severe family disruptions and negative economic effects.

Chronic age-related disease patients (CARDs) often end up in intermediate care units or specialized centers in order to recover from vascular accidents such as strokes, heart attacks and kidney failures, while others may experience motor disability caused by bone and joint injuries. These events often lead to falls, dementia and incontinence that can prompt long term institutionalization.

Fortunately, most health professionals believe that a person who is overweight or obese can significantly improve their health and well-being by losing at least 10% of body weight, as long as the person avoids gaining it back. In conclusion, in order to live a healthy and better life, it is essential for those who are overweight or obese to lose weight.

It must be pointed out that for the very obese patient, exercise is not an effective method to reduce weight because the body is very efficient in converting nutrients into energy, i.e. *several hours of vigorous exercise is equivalent* only *to a small dessert.* Moreover, despite its benefits, exercise can be rather risky in the obese, as it may cause accidents and even trigger degenerative arthritis.

Exercise in obese individuals should be moderate at the beginning and only after having a significant weight loss; patients may be progressively exercised in order to achieve a *greater oxygen consumption capacity*. This increased capacity is reflected in a lower heart frequency (registered upon awakening) and minimal tachycardia with exercise.

It is important to underscore that physical exercise, even in elderly patients, can indeed produce muscular hypertrophy (increased strength), improve coordination, reduce the risk of falls and diminish coronary risk. Although during exercise the coronary risk increases, it has been concluded that coronary accidents during exercise are not very frequent; furthermore, this possibility can be evaluated by exercise testing.

Hippocrates, called the Father of Western Medicine, wisely coined the following phrases:

"Men dig their graves with their own teeth."

"Let food be your medicine and medicine be your food".

Controlling and moderating appetite, along with understanding and monitoring the biological, psychological and social impacts of obesity and its consequences, should again become the central pillar of medicine.

Jaime Durand, MD

EMOTIONAL HUNGER

Food, for many people, does more than satisfy their hunger: it comforts their emotions. When they become calm or soothe feelings by eating they are "eating emotionally". This behavior is one of the most common causes of weight gain and obesity.

Eating only when you are truly hungry seems a simple and obvious recommendation. However, it is the dietary advice most difficult to follow. Why? Because of the previous lifestyle conditioning and emotional baggage each individual carry.

Signs of emotional hunger

True physical hunger is a complex psychophysical response to low energy reserves aimed to correct low blood sugar. True physical hunger does not seek a "sugar high".

There are several behavioral differences that distinguish emotional hunger and physical hunger:

1. Emotional hunger comes suddenly, while true hunger happens gradually.

2. When you are eating something specific to fill a void that is not related to hunger, you are feeling emotional hunger. For example, longing for a specific food such as pizza, ice cream, chocolate ...when you are really hungry, you will accept many other options.

3. Emotional hunger needs to be filled immediately with a particular food. Physical hunger can wait.

4. If you're eating to calm an emotional need, it is likely you will continue eating even if you feel satisfied. If you eat because you are really hungry it is easier to quit when you feel satisfied.

5. Emotional hunger can be accompanied by feelings of guilt; with true hunger, eating is a pleasure.

How to overcome emotional hunger

Recognizing the difference between emotional hunger and real hunger is the key to eating food within healthy parameters. It is necessary not only to observe and know why and how you eat, but it is useful to keep track of the foods you eat and how you feel about eating them.

- Do not eat because of boredom, unhappiness, tension, stress or other emotional reason.
- Determine whether you are really hungry. If the answer is "not sure," then you are not.
- Avoid eating quickly or in a hurry or while you are working, watching TV, etc.
- Postpone mealtime if not hungry.

Wait until a genuine natural desire to eat comes to you. Before you eat, take some time to practice any activity you like or distract yourself with some work to do, reading, gardening or better, take a walk. The performance of some regular physical activity is the best way to foster true hunger and to control anxiety.

It is important not to rush weight loss. Being in a hurry breeds anxiety. Avoid strict diets that only lead to states of compulsion and lack of motivation. Find encouragement in achieving positive changes in your eating habits.

Characteristic signs of "true" hunger without being in a prolonged fasting

- Mouth salivation
- Mind optimistic, clear and happy (however, sometimes anger)
- Hunger that persists even if you wait for the meal

Characteristic signs of false hunger

- Dry mouth, thick tongue, bad breath
- Stomach twinges
- Cramps, aches and nausea
- Hunger sensation that disappears with waiting

Some tips to apply

During the day, drink plenty of hot or cold **liquids**: water, broth, green tea, hot tea, natural fruit juices and lemonade.

Include in each meal **foods** with an adequate supply of fiber, prepared so as to prolong the digestive process and generate the satiety sensation.

A useful resource to control anxiety and keep you on track with eating healthy foods is to blend yourself a smoothie with 1 medium banana and 1 / 2 cup of skim milk. It is also helpful to prepare and have handy lemonade, nonfat yogurt or dietary gelatin with bits of fruit, and freeze it into ice cubes.

Techniques to avoid being tempted

Never skip breakfast. Be active after breakfast. It's a good strategy to start burning calories early in the mornings.

Eat several meals a day: learn to choose and measure what you eat, so you will stay satisfied for a longer time. Keep chicken broth or green tea in the fridge ready to use upon arriving at home after a busy day, or prepare some hot tea. Cool down; take a shower when you come back from work -- these routines will help you not to jump onto the fridge.

Avoid being near food longer than necessary. While cooking, have at hand a cup of hot soup with vegetables, bits of celery, carrot sticks, and diced tomatoes with basil or green apples. In this way you will have a full stomach and this will prevent you from tasting the food more than necessary. A light soup or a green leaves' salad before the main meal will be of great help to reduce appetite.

That an ingredient or food is considered low in fat does not mean you can eat it unconstrained. For example, if you eat a huge plate of mashed pumpkin, you will not lose weight. Instead of that, indulge yourself with a small portion of mashed potatoes without leaving aside your diet plan. If you live with someone else at home and there are tempting foods stored, place them in airtight boxes (even tape them), and put them out of your direct eyesight on higher shelves. Suggest someone else to take care of them.

There is no need to isolate one's self or to force the family to adopt your diet. You may modify some family recipes and enjoy delicious meals with fewer calories. Prepare various side dishes to accompany an entree. For example, if you prepared a baked chicken, you can accompany it with mixed vegetables for yourself, and with potatoes for the rest of the family.

When you decide to prepare pasta, you can enjoy it without increasing its calorie content if accompanied by a homemade tomato sauce or some sautéed vegetables. Avoid eating them with grated cheese. In preparing pizza, you may use fresh sliced tomato, sliced onions, sautéed peppers and small amounts of grated skim mozzarella. Virgin oils extracted from nuts, in adequate quantities, are a healthy choice.

Assign a single place to eat and avoid leaving food near beds or chairs. Bring the dishes served to the table: a dish full of food is a temptation hard to control. Let your eating utensils rest on the table between bites, especially when you are eating high calorie foods.

Avoid spending too much time at the table after meals: family meetings can be done without having enticing meals. Love has nothing to do with eating a lot. Sometimes we try to express love by providing a large meal to our loved ones but this is a cultural phenomenon.

Do not promise you will not eat a candy again. Propose yourself a reasonable limit, "once or twice a week." If you choose to indulge yourself, while doing it, dedicate the time and space it deserves. If you eat fast, your craving for something delicious will remain simmering. Chew slowly and enjoy food with your eyes closed, this will make you eat less.

Do not be discouraged when you are not able to control your appetite: the fact that it is hard for you to lose weight does not mean you're not reaching your goal. Find other satisfactions that contribute to not live so attentive to what you should not eat. To be patient and overcome barriers is part of the evolutionary process that will lead to a healthy life.

The best way to lose weight is to reduce your intake. However, it is recommended to increase your caloric expenditure by doing exercise. To do this, simply take a walk every day, climb stairs, dance at home or do your chores with more energy. Another option is to take care of a dog, who will force you to take him for a walk several times a day.

Eating out

If you have to be many hours without eating anything, take in a good amount of liquids between meals. If occasionally you want a serving of strawberries, apple or a fruit salad, we recommend you to ingest them always separated from the main meals.

When you feel like eating something that can cause weight gain, share the portion and accompany it with a salad or vegetables with lemon. When choosing vegetables for a salad, remember cabbage and summer squash or zucchini have half the calories of carrots, tomatoes, beetroot or beet, and squash. Therefore, you can eat twice the amount of the first without fear of gaining weight.

Special occasions

Do not fast before or after going to a party. Give yourself a tacit permission to eat a bit of everything. However, eat a light snack before the occasion. When you serve an appetizer, add cherry tomatoes, mushrooms with garlic and parsley, heart of palm, celery sticks, raw carrots and low fat cheese. In this way, you can avoid high-calorie snacks.

If you wish to drink alcohol, prefer dry champagne or wine, always in moderation. Remember that sweeter or higher alcohol content the beverage has, the more calories it provides.

Once at the party avoid the first tray since it's unlikely you will get something light. Besides, once you start eating flour, it could become impossible to contain yourself from eating the rest of the food. Instead, choose cheeses, lean meats and salads, if any. Remove sauces and control the side dishes for the main dish.

Eat in moderation so you can choose a small portion of dessert. If you are going to enjoy an ice cream with your family, prefer one prepared with water and fruit instead of cream, which contains twice the amount of calories. Consuming fruit, yogurt and lots of fluids will help you to recover your healthy regimen if you have eaten more than what you should.

Note: You can use blends of natural herbs to eliminate liquids retention. However, before using them, consult with your doctor.

Medical note:

The struggle of hunger during a prolonged low calorie regimen requires effort and tenacity. The patient has to have a good night sleep complying with the recommended hours of sleep time that is required to repair lean body mass (muscle) during deep sleep. If this is not accomplished during a dieting period this tissue is lost.

A recent scientific experiment done at the University of Birmingham in the United Kingdom had the objective of determining if inadequate sleep curtailed the weight loss efficacy of hypo caloric diets in obese patients and determined that: In comparison to patients that slept 8.5 hours, the patients that slept 5.5 hours loss 60 % more muscle mass and had 55 % less adipose tissue loss as well as reporting feeling more hungry and having a metabolic state that consumed less adipose tissue.

The success of a healthy living program depends on

- ***desiring it as one's own lifestyle***
- ***understanding it and being able to practice it***
- ***testing its effectiveness in the short and long term***

What is a calorie?

A **calorie** is the amount of heat required to raise the temperature of 1 gram of water, one degree Celsius.

The calories contained in food are equal to the energy the body can get from them. This energy can be found in the fats, sugars and proteins in food.

These three nutritional elements are transformed among themselves thanks to the cellular machinery (enzymes) whose design is contained in our genes, located in the inherited DNA.

Why does weight gain happen?

Weight gain happens when calories consumed in meals and beverages exceed calories required for **basal metabolism** and **physical activity**. This calories excess is stored in fatty tissue and obesity develops.

Basal metabolism is the minimum amount of energy required to survive breathing.

Food, its properties and benefits

Food is a substance (solid or liquid) ingested by living organisms to satisfy appetite, physiological functions, regulate metabolism, physical activity and maintain body temperature. Foods contain proteins, lipids, carbohydrates, minerals, vitamins and water.

Proteins
Proteins are complex organic compounds containing nitrogen, carbon, oxygen and hydrogen, whose basic structure is a chain of amino acids.

Amino Acids
Amino acids are organic substances with an acid and an amine function, which is the basis of proteins. In other words, they are the constituent elemental units of molecules called proteins.

Amino acids are classified into two groups:

Essential amino acids: are those that the body can not produce and must be supplied by food. These amino acids include, for example, cysteine (containing sulfur), lysine (necessary for collagen) and tryptophan (the scarcest in the body) which provide aromatic rings for the biochemistry of the body.

These essential amino acids are found in milk, cheese, eggs, mushrooms and meat (fish, shellfish, birds, mammals, etc.). A single source of protein does not contain all essential amino acids.

To obtain all the different essential amino acids the body requires, it is necessary the ingestion of varied sources of protein. Therefore, it is necessary to alternate our consumption of the different high protein containing foods. We also find essential proteins in legumes, vegetables, nuts, grains, fruits, etc.

It is important to point out that pure vegetarian diet is insufficient for the survival of human populations. This is due to the scarce content of some of the essential amino acids (lysine, for example) and to the smaller biological value of protein in vegetables (compared to meat). There have been fatal accidents in people who followed diets based on a single protein source.

Biological value is a measure of the proportion of absorbed protein from a food which becomes incorporated into the proteins of the organism's body. **The biological value of protein from different protein food sources can be measured as the relative ability of the diverse food (containing protein) to increase the weight of growing animals**.

Medical Note: The biological value of animal protein sources is 100%, more than double the biological value of vegetable proteins. For example, wheat biological value is about 38%.

The cheese whey protein has a biological value even higher than beef, given its high absorption by the body. It represents an ideal source of amino acids for those who need a nutritious high nitrogen diet.

Usually, it is consumed about one gram of protein per kilogram of body weight per day. Excessive intake of protein, above 1.5 g. per kg body weight per day, is not recommended because the nitrogen excess in the body produces acidification, with consequent erosion of constituent structures (bones, muscles, etc.).

Medical Note: increased protein intake may be indicated in critical medical conditions.

Nonessential amino acids are produced by the body from essential amino acids, as well as from sugars and fats. Examples of nonessential amino acids are aspartic acid, glutamic acid and glycine.

Selective use of some of these amino acids is associated with the consumption of fats and depends on whether the individual is in a prolonged fast (voluntary or involuntary) or not. There are the ketogenic amino acids, which can not be converted into glucose (used in the "ketogenic diet" to control severe intractable epilepsy); or the glucogenic amino acids that can be converted into glucose.

All proteins are made up of chains of amino acid molecules. The specific sequence of the different amino acids that constitute all proteins, are encoded in inherited DNA. Proteins can be **enzymes** (catalysts, organic chemical accelerators that transform nutrients) or **constitutive** proteins (which make up the tissues cellular structure).

Amino acids are molecules containing nitrogen that are obtained from the food protein that we eat. The proteins are digested - broken or decomposed - into amino acids by the intestinal juices. These amino acids are then reconstituted inside the intestinal cells forming other proteins, which are characteristic of the new organism's cells.

These body proteins carry out a number of functions in all living organism. The **constitutive** proteins are necessary for the **construction and repair** of muscles, bones, tissues, blood and organs. The **enzymatic** proteins are necessary to catalyze (accelerate) the body's biochemical reactions (metabolism) in order to modify molecules and thus harness the energy contents of fats, sugars, and proteins.

This enzymatic activity allows energy transformation from nutrients (sugars, fats and amino acids) into an **energy "coin" molecule** called ATP, which happens to be the "currency" of cellular energy. This "energy currency" is used to carry out all of the body activities.

Enzymes are manufactured to fit the body's needs at a particular time and / or at different life history periods (childhood, adolescence, adulthood and old age). Thus, the same body has different proportions of sugars, fats or proteins during their different life periods, always according to the genetic program that determines its history. For example, as individuals grow older they have increasingly more fat, less protein (less muscle) and less water in their body.

The **constituent** proteins of the body are those that form part of cell walls and of tissues fibers that constitute the interstitial tissue (e.g. collagen), tendons, muscles, bones and so on.

The **sequence of different amino acids in proteins** (either **constitutive** or **enzymatic**) is encoded by the inherited DNA, unlike the **sequence of sugars or lipids of biological molecules in the body, that are not encoded in inherited DNA**.

The **sequence** of different sugars (that makes up complex carbohydrates) or the **sequence of lipids** (that makes up complex fats) is not encoded by inherited DNA. The sequence of lipids and complex sugars in the body is dependent on the activities of the diverse protein enzymes, responsible for the glycosylation or the addition of lipids to other biological molecules in the body.

Depending on their source, dietary proteins are of vegetable or animal origin. The first type can be found in vegetables, soybeans, grains, dry fruits or legumes, and the second in animals: red and white meats, fish, shellfish, eggs, milk and mushrooms.

Fats
Fats are organic compounds consisting of carbon, hydrogen and oxygen (do not contain nitrogen), and are the major source of energy derived from food and stored in the body.

Fats belong to a group of substances called lipids, and come in liquid or solid form.

Among the three nutrients in the body, fat is the one that provides the most calories per gram of food. Fats provide 9 calories of energy per gram of weight, while sugars and proteins provide 4 calories per gram of weight.

The fat used for feeding is a triglyceride, made up of 3 long fatty acids bonded to a short glycerol molecule.

Fatty acids may be essential and nonessential:

Essential fatty acids such as linoleic acid (omega 6) and linolenic acid (omega 3) can not be produced by the body and must be obtained directly from food. They are important for controlling inflammation, blood clotting and development of brain and nervous tissue.

Non-essential fatty acids, such as oleic acid, palmitic acid, etc., serve primarily as a source of energy (working capacity), and is stored in the adipose tissue like other fats.

Fats that accumulate in the adipose cells (of the adipose tissue) can also help protect the body from temperature changes in the environment (outdoors).

It is important to point out that accumulated fat usage occurs during a prolonged fast as well as after twenty minutes of exercising, when the carbohydrates from glycogen (accumulated sugar in the liver) have been consumed. Then the organism begins to depend from the calories derived from the lipids of fat.

Fats (**lipids or triglycerides**) can contain chains of saturated fatty acids (saturated with hydrogen) or partially saturated, the so called "unsaturated fatty acids" (as there are no completely unsaturated fats).

Saturated Fat
Saturated fats constitute the most consumed worldwide lipid type. They have no double bonds between the carbons of their fatty acid chain and most of them are solid at body temperature.

These fats are found in animal products: butter, cheese, whole milk, ice cream, milk cream and fatty meats. They are also found in some vegetable oils: coconut oil, palm oil, peanut oil and cottonseed oil.

"Unsaturated fats"
These are fats that have double-bonds in their carbon fatty acid chain (as well a less hydrogen content) and are more flexible than saturated fats (lower melting point).

Being more flexible, their cell membranes are more liquid but chemically more reactive, i.e. become rancid or oxidized more easily in the absence of antioxidants like vitamin E. However, their flexibility allows a better flow of biological components (fewer blood clots) and help lower blood cholesterol. Contain the same amount of calories as saturated fats and are mostly found in vegetable oils.

There are two types of "unsaturated fats":

- Monounsaturated fats: olive, avocado and extra virgin palm or raw oils.
- Polyunsaturated fats: sunflower, sesame, safflower, corn, linseed, almonds, walnuts, other dry fruits, grapes, soybeans, *sacha inchi*, among other extra virgin or raw oils.

Cis-monounsaturated fatty acids:
These fatty acids are naturally present in the vast majority of animal and vegetable fat.

Animal fats have higher saturated oils than vegetable oils. Cow's milk has only small amounts of trans oils. Vegetable fat from palm and coconut have saturated oils. Vegetables oils from olive, avocado and palm have lots of cis-monounsaturated fat.

Trans-monounsaturated fatty acids:
These fatty acids are formed when vegetable oil hardens due to an artificial hydrogenation process to make margarine, in order that it can be stored longer without becoming rancid.

Trans-monounsaturated fat (margarine) is more rigid than saturated fat. Neither of them melt readily at body temperature (98.6 ° F - 37 ° C, or in the mouth) and both remain solid inside the body. Moreover, this Trans fat can raise levels of LDL (bad cholesterol), as well as lower the HDL (good cholesterol), increasing the risk of atherosclerosis (stiffness and obstruction of the arteries). These trans fatty acids are also found in fried fast food and some commercial products which have been processed to become crispy. Among them are margarines, biscuits, crackers and other foods of prolonged storage.

Natural cis-monounsaturated acids do not have the negative properties of **trans monounsaturated fatty** and a watchful consumer must know to distinguish them. This means that a product with the same amount of monounsaturated oil may contain different amounts of the trans or cis form. Currently, it is mandatory to consign this information on the labels of products that are sold.

Animal fats and butter contain a very small amount of vitamin E, so they quickly become rancid (oxidize).

It is recommended to eat vegetables of different colors every day to consume these antioxidants, which exist abundantly in plants to protect themselves from the oxygen they produce.

Vegetable oils contain vitamin E in a natural way, most notably, wheat germ, corn, sunflower, cottonseed and palm oils.

Hydrogenated or saturated fats and partially hydrogenated or "unsaturated fats"

Hydrogenated fats are oils that have been hardened, such as margarine. In partially hydrogenated fats, oils have hardened to some extent. Foods made with hydrogenated oils should be avoided because they contain high levels of trans fatty acids. (It is recommended to read ingredients on the food label).

Note on cholesterol

Cholesterol in food, as well as cholesterol produced by the body, serves for the constitution of cell membranes and the formation of sex hormones.

Animal fats, egg yolks, shellfish and butter contain high concentrations of cholesterol. Patients with high cholesterol should avoid these foods.

Polyunsaturated fat

These are the omega 9 (oleic acid) that can be produced by the human body from unsaturated fats as well as from the other polyunsaturated fats like the essential oil omega 6 (linoleic acid) and omega 3 (linolenic acid).

The biological effects of omega 9 are usually interposed by their interactions with fatty acids omega 3 and omega 6. Omega 6 fats are derivatives of linoleic acid. It is recommended to eat moderately this essential fatty acid, whose activity partially counter opposes the antithrombotic beneficial activity of omega-3.

Omega-3 fats are important due to its derivatives EPA and DHA. These two biologically active fatty acids are produced by the plankton from the cold waters of the Polar Regions. They are extremely flexible and do not freeze, allowing photosynthesis in algae.

These oils that accumulate in fishes that feed on these algae (phytoplankton) are immensely beneficial to the human body because they prevent inflammatory processes, reduce triglyceride and blood fats, and stimulate neural development.

However, big fishes, which are the end of the ocean's food chain, are accumulating mercury and PCBs (harmful chemicals) too. Through other mechanisms, these toxic substances decrease the protective effect of EPA and DHA, so it is not recommended to eat frequently large fish such as swordfish, shark, king mackerel, tilefish, and so on.

Avoid eating large fish is especially important for pregnant women who should not eat fish more than twice a week. The general population must alternate various small fish to avoid the accumulation of mercury and PCB.

The human body also produces small amounts of EPA and DHA from essential linolenic acid omega-3. That is why pregnant women should supplement this essential oil ingesting a diet rich in virgin vegetable oils containing a large amount of omega 3. These polyunsaturated oils are essential for fetal development. Use organic unprocessed ("omega flow process" - see product label) flaxseed, soybean, peanut, rapeseed oils as sources of Omega 3 oil. A virgin olive and flaxseed oil mix is ideal.

The oily products that contain the highest amount of omega 6 are sunflower, soybean, corn, cotton seeds and dry fruits, among other oils. Those that contain fewer amount of omega 6 are palm, coconut, olive, avocado and linseed virgin oil, as well as butter, meat fat and lard. High intake of omega 6 oils has been linked to breast and possibly prostate cancers. Inedible oils include processed linseed, tung, and castor.

Carbohydrates

Carbohydrates are a category of foods that includes sugars, starches and fiber. The main function of carbohydrates is to supply energy to the body, especially the brain and nervous system. They also serve for the making up of glycoprotein (sugar-coated proteins that allow a specific function).

Complex carbohydrates, contained in foods of animal and vegetable origin, are in the form of glycogen, starch, maltose, lactose and sucrose. These are broken down in the intestine into glucose, fructose and galactose to be absorbed, metabolized (inter converted) and stored as glycogen in the liver and muscles. Finally, they are used to produce fast energy from the glucose derived from glycogen or from the glucose that has been ingested.

Carbohydrates are classified as simple (monosaccharide), semi-simple (disaccharide) or complex. This classification depends on the chemical structure of the food source they come from and is associated with the speed with which the sugar is digested and absorbed. Simple carbohydrates have one (single) or two (semi-simple) sugars, while complex carbohydrates have three or more sugar in their chain.

Simple sugars are fructose (found in fruit sucrose), galactose (found in lactose present in dairy products) and glucose (found in maltose and other disaccharides).

Double or semi-simple sugars include lactose (found in dairy products), maltose (found in certain vegetables and in beer) and sucrose (found, for example, in cane sugar). Honey, unlike table sugar, has small amounts of double sugars. It's mainly glucose and fructose and contains a small amount of vitamins and minerals.

Complex carbohydrates, often called "rich in starch" food, include:

- breads and cereals
- starchy vegetables
- legumes

Semi-simple carbohydrates, that contain vitamins and minerals found naturally in:

- fruits
- milk and its derivatives
- vegetables

Simple carbohydrates are also found in processed and refined sugars such as:

- sweets
- table sugar
- syrups
- regular carbonated drinks (not diet), such as soda

It is not advisable to eat sweets or processed or refined sugars (pure glucose) as they can cause tooth decay (caries) and diabetes.

Glucose enters the cells through the action of the hormone insulin, secreted by the pancreas after a meal rich in sugars. If sugars consumed are simple, its absorption is rapid and insulin secretion is violent, so it is recommended the use of complex sugar foods. This is particularly true for diabetic patients.

In diabetics, the **production** or **use** of insulin is defective depending on whether they have diabetes type 1 or type 2, respectively. In diabetics type I (juvenile or thin) insulin production is insufficient and this leads to high glucose levels in blood, since the main function of insulin is the entry of glucose from blood into cells.

In diabetics type II (obese) the **use** of insulin is inadequate, since the large amount of fat in the body presents a high number of insulin receptors in relation to the amount of insulin normally produced by the pancreas. This imbalance or relative deficiency of insulin causes high blood glucose levels, despite paradoxically high insulin levels in blood because the pancreas secretes insulin trying to offset the high number of insulin receptors in the body.

The reason why diabetes affects the body is due to damage incurred in the absence of sugar inside the cell, as well as its excess in blood. The lack of intracellular sugar produces metabolic changes that cause diabetic acidosis, which if not controlled leads to death.

High levels of blood sugar promote an accelerated link **with** proteins (spontaneous process, non-enzymatic) and produce advanced glycosylation proteins in these patients (AGE). These body proteins extensively glycosylated are aging markers of cells and tissues, and are the cause of body damage to the nervous level (eyes), kidney and cardiovascular system.

The measurement and monitoring of these highly glycosylated proteins (e.g. hemoglobin A1c or glycohemoglobin), serve to improve the treatment for diabetes. Hemoglobin A1C, representing the average blood sugar over the past 3 months, allows the physician to adjust more precisely the dose of anti-diabetic / anti-glycemic agents.

The consumption of simple sugars is not recommended because it is associated with the development of obesity, atherosclerosis and metabolic disease (high triglycerides). Therefore, it is convenient to avoid soft drinks.

Vitamins: are essential organic substances that the body can not produce. Their nature and composition are varied. They function as enzymatic co-factors and promote catalysis or acceleration of metabolism's chemical reactions for the inter-conversion of sugars, fats and / or protein.

They are also components of constitutive pigments and/or other substances in the organism. Vitamins are essential in the metabolic processes that take place in the nutrition of living beings.

All vitamins have very specific functions on the body and must be included in the daily diet to prevent deficiencies. There is no magic food that contains all the vitamins: only the right combination of food groups can meet the requirements of all essential elements for life.

Only vitamin D can be produced in small amounts by the sun exposed skin. The rest of the vitamins are only obtained through food.

There are 13 essential vitamins necessary for the body to function. Vitamins are grouped into two categories:

- Fat-soluble vitamins, which are stored in fatty tissues of the body, allowing us to survive for some time without eating them.
- Water-soluble vitamins, which the body needs to eat regularly because they are used immediately and are not stored (vitamin B 12 is the exception).

- The **fat-soluble** are those that dissolve in fat, accumulate in the body (especially liver) and can be toxic if consumed in high doses. They come from foods rich in fat, and are also more resistant to cooking than water-soluble vitamins.

- Vitamin A (retinol) and animal foods (beta-carotene) from plant origin
- Vitamin D
- Vitamin E
- Vitamin K

- The **water-soluble** are those that dissolve in water and do not accumulate. They come from water-rich foods and generally are not toxic. Any excess water-soluble vitamin is excreted through urine.

- Vitamin C
- Vitamin B 1 (Thiamine)
- Vitamin B 2 (Riboflavin)
- Vitamin B 3 (Niacin)
- Vitamin B 5 (Pantothenic acid)
- Vitamin B 6 (Pyridoxine)
- Vitamin B 8 (Biotin)
- Vitamin B 9 (Folate or folic acid) mostly in the plant kingdom.
- Vitamin B 12 (Cyanocobalamin) of animal origin, since it is not found in vegetables.

Fat-soluble vitamins:

Vitamin A, which helps to form and maintain healthy teeth, bones, soft tissue, mucous membranes and skin.

Vitamin A is present in carotene (yellow vegetables), and in retinol (of animal origin). Good sources include:

- halibut oil
- apricot
- cod
- yellow yam
- meat
- cream
- eggs
- liver
- milk
- mango
- butter
- seafood
- melon
- fish
- red pepper
- cheese
- kidneys
- leafy green vegetables
- carrot
- pumpkin

Vitamin D, also known as the "sunshine vitamin" because the body produces it up after exposure to sunlight. Ten to fifteen minutes of sun exposure three times a week is enough to supply the body's requirement of this vitamin, but in older people this may be insufficient.

This vitamin promotes the absorption of calcium in the body, essential for the development and maintenance of healthy teeth and bones. It also helps maintain adequate blood levels of calcium and phosphorus.

Normally, milk is supplemented with vitamin D to prevent rickets (vitamin D deficiency) in the population.

Vitamin D. Good sources include:

- cereals
- cream
- fortified milk
- butter
- margarine
- oysters
- fish
- cheese
- egg yolk

Vitamin E, also known as tocopherol, which plays an important role in the formation of red blood cells and helps the body use vitamin K.

Vitamin E. Good sources include:

- raw vegetable or extra virgin oils
- olives
- asparagus
- spinach and other leafy green vegetables
- wheat germ
- eggs
- corn
- nuts
- seeds

Vitamin K, that is important for blood clotting and bone formation. It is present in vegetables despite being a fat-soluble vitamin. For this reason, patients who are taking anticoagulants, such as Coumadin (Warfarin), should keep a diet with the same amount of vegetables (no matter how much or little, but always the same amount) to prevent the occurrence of bleeding or thrombosis due to excess or inhibition, respectively, of the Coumadin. In other words, the dose of Coumadin is regulated according to the consumption of a steady diet of vegetables, not vice versa.

Vitamin K. Good sources include:

- apricot
- peas
- celery
- broccoli
- cereals
- cauliflower
- cabbage
- asparagus
- spinach
- pear
- soybeans
- grape
- leafy green vegetables
- carrot

Water-soluble vitamins:

Vitamin B1 or **thiamine**, which helps the body cells convert carbohydrates into energy. It is essential for proper functioning of heart and maintenance of nerve cells.

Alcoholic patients require this vitamin to avoid toxicity of alcohol, likewise, is required by patients who are taking glucose supplements.

Vitamin B 1. Good sources include:

- peas
- lean meats
- dry beans
- fruits and vegetables
- wholegrain
- enriched breads, cereals and pasta
- fish
- dairy products
- soybeans

Vitamin B2 or **riboflavin**, which works in conjunction with other B complex vitamins and plays an important role in body growth and red blood cell production. It is essential for good function of eyes and metabolism of carbohydrates, fats and proteins.

Vitamin B 2. Good sources include:

- lean meat
- eggs
- milk and dairy products
- legumes
- nuts
- breads and cereals, often fortified with riboflavin
- vegetables

Vitamin B3, or **niacin**, a B complex vitamin, that helps to maintain healthy skin and nerves. Also has lowering effects on triglycerides and increases HDL (good cholesterol). It is also vital for converting food into energy. This vitamin is very important in the use of tryptophan (which is the scarcest amino acid of the body), and is necessary for the formation of serotonin, (primary sleep inducer when enters the brain by means of insulin). Sugar induces insulin, allowing the entry of tryptophan into the brain, which is why a glass of milk with sugar helps to sleep.

Niacin B 3. Good sources include:

- artichoke
- peas
- lean meats
- red meat
- cereals and enriched breads
- eggs
- legumes
- nuts
- fish
- chicken
- dairy products
- leafy green vegetables
- carrot

Vitamin B5, or pantothenic acid, essential for the metabolism of food, plays an important role in the production of hormones and cholesterol.

Vitamin B 5. Good sources include:

- avocado
- broccoli and other vegetables of cabbage family
- lean beef
- wholegrain cereals
- dry fruits
- eggs
- legumes
- lentils
- yeast
- potato and sweet potato
- pear
- fish
- dairy products

Vitamin B6, also known as **pyridoxine**, helps the immune system to produce the antibodies needed to fight many diseases. Furthermore, this vitamin helps maintain nerve function normal, and form red blood cells. The body uses it to help break down proteins: the higher is protein intake, the greater the need to ingest vitamin B 6.

Vitamin B 6 (pyridoxine). Good sources include:

- poultry
- sweet potato
- red meat
- cereals
- dry fruits
- liver
- potato
- fish
- banana
- egg yolk

Vitamin B8 or **biotin** is essential for the metabolism of proteins and carbohydrates, as well as for the production of hormones and cholesterol.

Vitamin B 8. Good sources include:

- broccoli and other vegetables of cabbage family
- lean beef
- wholegrains
- eggs
- legumes
- yeast
- potato and sweet potato
- fish

- dairy products

Folate, which works with vitamin B12 to form red blood cells, is necessary for the production of DNA and controls tissue growth, as well as cell function.

Every pregnant woman should make sure she gets adequate amounts of this vitamin, due to the fact that low levels of folate are associated with birth defects in babies such as Spina Bifida.

Many foods (cereals) are now fortified with folic acid. If folic acid supplementation becomes necessary to treat anemia, it is essential that the patient has normal B12 levels to prevent a neuropathy.

To prevent congenital malformations of the central nervous system of fetuses, cereals today are supplemented with folic acid. Pregnant women should make sure that cereals they eat are fortified with this vitamin.

Vitamin B 9 (folic acid or folate). Good sources include:
- cabbage
- cauliflower
- orange juice
- lentils
- leafy green vegetables

Vitamin B 12, or cyanocobalamin, which is important in metabolism, like other B complex vitamins, contributes to the formation of red blood cells and maintenance of the central nervous system.

Vitamin B 12 is the only water-soluble vitamin that can be stored in the liver for many years.

Vitamin B 12 (cyanocobalamin). Good sources include:
- red meat
- eggs
- milk and dairy products
- seafood
- chicken

Because vitamin B 12 is the largest vitamin, its absorption requires special proteins in the stomach (intrinsic factor) and a functional terminal small intestine (ileum). Patients with mal-absorption of vitamin B12 need regular injections of this product to avoid developing pernicious anemia.

Vitamin C, also called ascorbic acid, is an antioxidant essential for healthy teeth and gums. This vitamin helps the body absorb iron and maintain healthy tissue, and also contributes to wound healing.

Vitamin C (ascorbic acid). Good sources include:

- broccoli
- citrus fruits and juices
- cabbage
- asparagus
- spinach
- strawberry
- cantaloupe melon
- mango
- turnips and other vegetables
- potato
- sweet potato
- pepper
- pineapple
- tomato
- fresh vegetables
- tomato
- vegetales frescos

Most other fruits and vegetables contain some vitamin C; fish and milk contain small amounts.

FIBER:

Dietary fiber is the part of plants that can not be digested. It includes the outer shell (bran) of cereals, pectin from apples, peel and fibrous parts of fruits and vegetables.

A diet low in fiber, combined with the consumption of fat and calories, can lead to obesity, constipation and diverticulitis. It is recommended to consume wheat or cereals wholegrain products, as they provide fiber to the body and reduce heart disease risk.

The fiber can be classified into soluble and insoluble, according to its affinity with water.

Soluble fiber mainly slows the glucose absorption, lowers blood cholesterol levels and is fermented by colonic bacteria, without a laxative effect.

Soluble fiber. Good sources include:

- some fruits and vegetables
- peas
- oats
- barley
- kidney bean

- lentils
- nuts
- seeds

Insoluble fiber, on the contrary, has mainly a laxative effect: accelerates intestinal transit and increases stool weight. It also reduces the absorption of glucose.

Insoluble fiber. Good sources include:
- wholegrain
- wheat bran
- vegetables

WATER:

Water is the principle of all living organisms. It is present in body cells and helps all body functions. For being the substance that can absorb (or lose) more heat without changing its temperature it regulates body temperature. Drinking water helps to reduce fever.

Water is vital for humans. To maintain health, it is essential to adopt habits that facilitate fluid intake. The human body does not accumulate more water than necessary; hence, the amount lost each day should be restored to ensure the smooth functioning of the body.

Adequate water consumption decreases bladder cancer, especially in smokers.

MINERALS:

Minerals are essential micro inorganic nutrients that form part of an organ or element of the body, such as bones or blood. They are obtained through all fruits, vegetables and other foods.

Minerals keep the cells of each body organ healthy and working properly. They also activate enzymes and help carry out several vital processes, such as breathing, digestion and blood stream circulation.
Minerals are part of fruits, vegetables and other foods. Although present in minute amounts, their content is sufficient for the needs of human beings.

The following, are among the most important for the body:

Iron **Magnesium** **Calcium** **Phosphorus** **Cobalt**

Selenium **Potassium** **Sodium** **Iodine** **Fluoride** **Zinc**

Iron
Used to produce hemoglobin and carry oxygen throughout the body. Its lack causes anemia, fatigue and depression; its excess favors infection and cirrhosis.

Iron is found in:

- birds
- red meat
- cereals
- dates
- dry fruits
- figs
- legumes
- sardines
- green leafy vegetables
- egg yolk

Magnesium

Helps in the functioning of muscles, in maintaining healthy bones, teeth and joints. Magnesium reduces cardiovascular disease. Its absence causes problems in muscles and nerves, causing weakness and seizures. Alcoholics or patients taking diuretics should take supplement of magnesium in their diet.

Magnesium is found in:

- almonds
- oat
- brown sugar
- red meat
- beans
- wheat germ
- figs
- corn
- nuts
- whole grains
- green leafy vegetables

Calcium

It is important for the formation and care of the bones and teeth. Involved in blood clotting, helps muscle function and is necessary for the nervous system. Its lack causes softening and muscle weakness, rickets, osteoporosis, promotes tooth decay and weak nails. Older people require more calcium in the diet. Calcium supplementation has proved beneficial. Low calcium in blood produces muscle contractures.

Calcium is found in:

- watercress
- green leafy vegetables
- milk
- butter
- parsley
- fish

- cheese
- sardines
- sesame seeds

Phosphorus
It is important for building bones and teeth. It regulates activity and metabolism of cells. Its lack causes weakness and anorexia.

Phosphorus can be found in:

- red meat
- cereals
- beans
- broad beans
- egg
- lentils
- seafood
- fish
- chicken
- cheese
- vegetables
- yogurt

Selenium
It is an antioxidant, protects against cancer, helps in proper functioning of the heart, liver and reproductive organs. It stimulates the immune system and assists in the functioning of the thyroid gland. Its lack causes muscle aches.

Selenium is found in:

- birds
- whole grains
- dry fruits
- milk
- tangerine
- seafood
- fish
- cheese
- vegetables

Potassium
Maintains the proper functioning and rate of the heart. It supports the transmission of nerve impulses and controls the level of body water. Its lack causes muscle weakness, fatigue, lack of energy and dizziness. Patients who are taking certain diuretics (such as Furosemide and Hydrochlorothiazide) lose potassium and may require supplementation of potassium (and magnesium), as these minerals are lost through urine. Patients with renal impairment (or who take diuretics such as Spironolactone or Ethacrynic Acid) should avoid taking potassium, since its accumulation can be fatal due to slowing of the heart (bradicardia).

Potassium is found in:

- asparagus
- fruit in general, especially banana
- milk
- melon
- potatoes
- green leafy vegetables

A decrease in potassium and/or iron causes fatigue. Patients with arrhythmias require maintaining normal potassium levels to prevent excitation of cardiac tissue. (Low blood potassium produces tachycardia and high blood potassium produces bradycardia).

Sodium
Serves for muscles and nerves function, regulates body fluids and helps digestion. Its lack causes dehydration, dizziness and low blood pressure.

It is preferable not to add salt to food to prevent hypertension. However, in elderly patients it may be required its supplementation when they develop low sodium blood levels. This is because of decreased sodium re-absorption, which is associated with kidney ageing.

Sodium is found in:

- olives
- smoked meat and fish
- cereals
- preserved and packaged food
- canned food
- dry fruits
- milk
- seafood
- bread
- fish
- cheese
- table salt

Iodine
Used by the thyroid to manufacture hormones thyroxine and triiodothyronine, which contain iodine. During childhood, iodine deficiency can cause cretinism, resulting in children's physical and mental retardation. Iodine deficiency causes goiter, a disease known by its abnormal enlargement.

Iodine is found in:

- seafood
- fish
- iodized table salt
- vegetables

Table salt is sold supplemented with iodine to prevent endemic goiter in the population.

Fluorine
It is useful in bone formation, providing them with greater resistance, as well as for the teeth, protecting them from decay. Their excess causes calcification of soft tissues and tooth staining.

Fluorine is found in:

- drinking water
- fruit
- seafood
- fish
- vegetables

In general, drinking water is supplemented with fluoride to prevent teeth decay.

During tooth brushing, if mouth rinses containing fluoride are used, the mouthwash should not be swallowed because fluorosis can occur (fluoride accumulation). Fluorosis causes soft tissue calcification and very calcified but fragile bones.

Zinc
Involved in metabolism of proteins and nucleic acids, stimulates the activity of approximately 100 enzymes and helps the immune system to function properly. It is necessary for wound healing, aids in the perceptions of taste and smell, in the synthesis of DNA and in the seminal gland activity.

Zinc is found in:

- peanuts
- red meat
- cereals
- dry fruits
- eggs
- legumes
- seafood
- sunflower seeds

The lack of zinc causes growth problems, infertility, decreased body's defenses, anemia, skin disorders and gradual loss of sensitivity of the senses of taste and smell.

Zinc should be supplemented in the elderly who are losing weight because they are not eating due to a decreased sensitivity to flavors. Stimulating taste contributes to weight regain.

OILS AND THEIR CONSUMPTION

The best known oils for human consumption are those obtained from:

Fruit:	olive, avocado and palm oil.
Legumes:	soybean, peanut.
Cereals:	corn and wheat seed germ or grain.
Dry fruits:	walnuts, almonds, hazelnuts, coconut and other dry fruits.
Other seeds:	sunflower, flaxseed, grapes, safflower, sesame, among others.

Olive Oil

Extra virgin olive oil is one of the Mediterranean diet pillars. This olive juice extracted from the olive tree (Olea europaea) is considered a healthy fat, mainly for its high content (76%) in oleic acid (monounsaturated) and low content in saturated fat. It also contains other components with antioxidant, anti-inflammatory, anti-thrombotic and anti-atherosclerotic properties.

It is important to buy a good quality extra virgin olive oil

You should be aware that the extra virgin oil is priced higher than other olive oils, to which usually are added extra virgin olive oil to sell it at higher prices as a pure extra virgin olive oil.

Extra virgin olive oil is a long life oil and has a high stability degree

In the kitchen, extra virgin olive oils are used to season fish, salads, cooked stews, legumes and other foods. Their strong flavor and aroma give foods a characteristic taste.

Avocado oil

Extra virgin avocado oil is extracted by cold pressing or centrifuging ripe avocado (*Persea americana*) pulp. This gourmet oil has in its composition about 85% of unsaturated fatty acids. Oleic acid is between 60 and 70%; linoleic acid varies between 9.8 and 15.6%; and palmitic acid, between 8.5 and 15.5%.

This oil is gentle to palate, rich in body and pleasant tasting; it does not stifle food taste, but rather enhances and heightens natural flavors of all preparations. It is delicious as a seasoning on salads and all kinds of vegetables, dressings or condiments for soups and fish.

Sunflower Oil

Sunflower oil is a vegetable oil extracted from the seeds of the sunflower plant (*Heliantus annus*). This cold-pressed oil contains vitamin E in large amounts, a 66% of linoleic acid (omega 6) and a 26% of monounsaturated oleic acid. The color of this oil is pale yellow and is characterized by its delicate flavor.

It is an alternative for those who prefer to dress their salads, vegetables and sauces with milder flavors.

Sesame Oil

Sesame oil also known as ajonjoli, is a vegetable oil derived from sesame seeds (*Sesamum indicum*),

The sesame seeds cultivated in India were the first oil source in mankind diet. Sesame oil contains between 35% and 50% polyunsaturated linoleic acid (omega 6), and between 35% and 50% monounsaturated oleic acid. Its composition includes zinc and a large amount of minerals.

The oil product from **toasted sesame seeds** -which in Asia is used both in Chinese and Korean cooking- has dark color and intense flavor. The oil coming from **untoasted sesame seeds** features a lighter color and a delicate flavor.

.

From a culinary point of view, the oil from toasted seeds grants a particular taste to bittersweet salads. Furthermore, it is a magnificent choice for accentuating the flavor of cooked foods before serving them.

Safflower Oil

Safflower or alazor oil is obtained from safflower seeds (*Carthamus tinetorius*), a plant native to India. The oil should be extracted in cold to maintain its extraordinary properties. **Safflower oil is perhaps the one with the greatest amount of essential fatty acids – 70% linoleic acid (omega 6) and 20% oleic acid.** It easily becomes rancid due to the natural composition of essential fatty acids it contains.

It is used in the kitchen as a dressing on salads and cooked legumes. This oil's hazelnut like aroma and flavor might be too intense. We suggest combining it with other milder tasting oils.

Corn Oil

Corn oil (Zea mays), is oil obtained by cold-pressed corn germ. It contains 59% of linoleic acid (omega 6) and 24% of monounsaturated oleic acid.

It is an important source of vitamin E, beneficial due to its therapeutic properties for the skin.

It has a mild and pleasant flavor and is used for dressing salads, vegetables and other foods.

Flaxseed Oil

Flaxseed oil is a vegetable oil extracted in cold from flax plant (*Linum usitatissimum*) seeds. Of all seed oils flaxseed oil is the one that contains the highest source (58%) of linolenic fatty acids (omega 3). It also contains 14% of linoleic acid (omega 6), in addition to 19% of monounsaturated oleic acid (omega 9). ***Alfa-linolenic fatty acids (omega 3) contained in flaxseed oil are the hardest to obtain and the most lacking in our diet.***

Flaxseed oil is deep orange-yellow and has a pleasant nut flavor. Used in raw vegetables salads, it offers an aromatic taste to legumes and other cooked foods.

Other Gourmet oils

Some of the healthy oils commercialized on a smaller scale, which are also recognized as ***gourmet oils,*** are those from ***almonds, hazelnuts, walnuts, macadamia nuts, among other dry fruits***. They are obtained by cold pressing and have the taste of the nut from which they come and some of them easily become rancid.

They are a tasty alternative for seasoning cooked vegetable, pasta or salads. Due to their intense flavor, we recommend to consume them in small dose, or to combine with other softer oils.

Grapeseed Oil

The ***grapeseed oil*** (Vitis vinifera) has a tenuous and subtle flavor, which is obtained from the pressed grape seeds. It contains approximately 70% linoleic acid. This oil is not much stable and must be stored in a container protected from light.

In the kitchen is often combined with other more concentrated and flavorful oils to obtain dressings with a more delicate flavor.

Sacha Inchi Oil

Sacha Inchi oil (*Plukenetia volubilis*) comes from a plant native to the Amazon region of Peru. It is obtained from selected seed by a cold pressing technique providing virgin oil. This oil is rich in omega 3 fatty acids (over 48%) and omega 6 (36%) and omega 9 (8%).

This oil is easy to digest and has a slight nutty flavor, which combined with balsamic vinegar gives a unique flavor to raw or cooked vegetables.

It has a limited production, gets rancid easily and once opened can only be refrigerated for 30 days.

Coconut oil is obtained from coconut pulp, the coconut palm (*Cocos nucifera*) fruit. It is solid at room temperature due to its high content of saturated fatty acids (88%).

The consumption of this oil is beneficial for patients with fats absorption problems. No bile is required for its venous intestinal assimilation. Digestion is facilitated because coconut oil contains a short-chain fatty acid, very soluble in water. In the other oils, the fat chain is longer, so the absorption is lymphatic and requires bile for digestion.

We recommend its use to add taste to vegetables or other foods. The use of this cooking oil is widely spread in some Caribbean countries.

Refined coconut oil is mainly used in food industry to produce cocoa butter and margarine substitutes in ice cream, cookies, sweets, bakery and other similar products.

Peanut oil comes from the peanut (*Arachis irypogaea*) seeds. **Virgin** peanut oil contains a significant proportion of linoleic acid (omega 6) as well as mono-unsaturated and poly- unsaturated fats. **Processed** peanut oil (or peanut butter) can contain trans oils and should be eaten with moderation.

It is important to point out that some people ***are allergic to peanuts, nuts or other dry fruits,*** so when they consume oils derived from these products, especially those cold extracted or unrefined, may suffer anaphylactic (allergic) accidents.

In order to choose the right oil we must bear in mind that the appropriate thing to do is to obtain extra virgin oils made from different natural sources. In fact, the consumption of different types of fats (monounsaturated, polyunsaturated and saturated) is adjusted in the body by metabolism if provided all different necessary nutrients.

Culinary suggestions for combining these oils:

Virgin oils are essential for the elaboration of dressings which go with salads and vegetables.

The most used formula for vinaigrettes is 3 parts of oil per 1 of acid (lemon or vinegar) *

* If you prefer it, you may vary the acid amount to taste

Dry fruits oils such as those made from walnuts, almonds or hazelnuts, perfectly combine with fruit vinegars, for example apple juice.

Gourmet oils containing some hot spicy flavor as chili, hot pepper or cayenne pepper, or those produced with some herbs like thyme or saffron, besides providing antioxidants are very tasty with white wine vinegars.

A classic dressing, which is a nice emulsion, is the one prepared with extra virgin olive oil and balsamic vinegar.

A nice bittersweet combination to dress vegetable salads containing fruits is that made of extra virgin olive oil, balsamic vinegar and honey.

If you wish a flavor not quite as strong, a bittersweet combination to dress salads is that made of extra virgin olive oil, bee honey and rice vinegar or "Mirin", delicately flavored and slightly sweet.

Other oils available in the market

Soybean oil is a light yellow oil obtained from soybeans (*Glycine max*). It is rich in unsaturated fats, of which 58% are polyunsaturated (especially Omega 3) and 23% are of monounsaturated acid.

Unrefined soybean oil has a delicate taste akin to herbs but when being stored often suffers unpleasant alterations due to oxidation. This oil is easily assimilated and digested.

Refined soybean oil is ***the most widely produced*** oil in the world, being the main countries producing it the U.S., Brazil and Argentina.

This oil is consumed ***refined*** in margarines, mayonnaise, salad dressings, frozen foods and commercial baked goods. Refined soybean oil is the main component of mixed oils, known as vegetable oils.

Canola oil is a vegetable oil obtained from varieties of turnip (*Brassica napus*) seeds.

One of the nations with a large production of this vegetable is Canada. In the decade 1960-70, Canada obtained an improved variety of this plant, which produced oils with very low levels of toxic substances (erucic acid). This is a different product to that derived from rapeseed.

Canola oil is widely used in the United States and Canada and, to a lower scale, in some European countries. The name ***canola*** is derived from ***Can****adian* ***o****il* ***l****ow* ***a****cid*, or Canadian oil low in acid. It has a low level of saturated fat and contains 30% linoleic acid (omega 6).

Refined corn oil is obtained from the germ of corn (*Zea mays*) using a chemical process of refinement. Yellow in color and mild flavor, tolerates high temperatures.

Refined corn oil is used for frying foods, in the elaboration of margarines, mayonnaise, consommés, and in the baking industry, among other processed foods.

Palm oil or **Red Crude Palm Oil,** due to its high carotenes content, is obtained by mechanical extraction of oil from the African palm fruit (*Elaeis guineensis*).

Refined palm oil is used in processed foods, frying oils, margarines, sauces, dressings, ice cream, cakes, cookies, etc.

It is the most produced in the world after refined soybean oil. Contains 45% of palmitic acid (saturated fatty acid), 5% of stearic acid (saturated fatty acid), 40% of oleic acid (monounsaturated fatty acid), and 10% of linoleic acid (polyunsaturated fatty acid).

Oils derived from modified or transgenic seeds are those industrial oils marketed under such names as "under linoleic, medium oleic" and "high oleic".

These terms are used to describe oils with a stable fatty acid composition during prolonged frying. Their costs are relatively low and are sold in large quantities. The most consumed transgenic oils are derived from corn, soybeans, canola, safflower and sunflower seeds. It is still unknown the biologic (and medical) outcome derived from these genetic alterations as they represent an evolutionary leap for the human immune system.

Refined vegetable oils combined are the result of mixing two or more oils from oilseeds.

Among the most common blends, there are those made from refined soybean oil, sunflower, cotton, corn germ, canola, safflower, peanut, and grape seed.

Additional information about oils and their metabolism

A **triglyceride** is the most common type of fat in nature. In practical terms, the total weight of any oil or margarine is made out of triglycerides. Each triglyceride molecule is made of three long (carbon) chain fatty acid molecules, each independently attached to the carbons of a shorter 3 carbon molecule called glycerin or glycerol. Each specific fatty acid consists of a variable, long string of carbon atoms.

Triglycerides are synthesized on the endoplasmic reticulum of all cells in the body. However it is in the liver parenchyma cells (hepatocytes) and in the adipose tissue cells where the process is more active and has metabolic relevance. Normally, after the fats have been digested in the small bowel, the intestinal cells allows the short chain free fatty acids to be absorbed directly through the venous blood, however the longer free fatty acids are re-synthesized and packaged into a lipoprotein denominated chylomicron.

These last lipoproteins go through the lymphatic system to eventually drain into the venous blood for them to reach the liver where they are processed. The liver then uses these triglycerides to make (adding cholesterol) the very low density lipoproteins (VLDL) that are secreted into the bloodstream to be used by the body becoming intermediate density lipoproteins (IDL) and then low density lipoproteins (LDL) returning to the liver as high density lipoproteins (HLD) to be finally used for bile production.

Because the liver is not an organ designed as a physiologic deposit for fat, all triglyceride accumulation is considered pathologic and called liver steatosis or fatty liver. On the contrary, the main function of the adipose tissue is the accumulation of triglycerides as a source of energy.

However the pathologic accumulation of fat in the adipose tissue, denominated obesity, is associated with a variety of endocrine and metabolic abnormalities that are under intense investigation, as they are thought to have causally a high impact in the contemporaneous population mortality. A small amount of triglycerides are normally kept in the skeletal and cardiac muscle for local use.

Triglycerides of different oils differ from each other due to the type of **fatty acids** they contain. There are three types of fatty acids, **saturated**, **monounsaturated** and **polyunsaturated**, depending if the molecule does not contain a double bond, contains one bond or contains 2 or more bonds, respectively.

The more **unsaturated** are the fatty acids of a triglyceride, the lower is their melting temperature, so they are more fluid (flexible) at room temperature or in the body. However, they become more reactive, i.e. less stable and more rancid. Thus, polyunsaturated fatty acids (linoleic and linolenic acid) are more reactive than mono-unsaturated fatty acids in a cis configuration (e.g., oleic acid).

The exception to this rule is that mono-unsaturated fatty acids with trans configuration (margarines) are stable but rigid fatty acids. Furthermore, as mentioned, they “do not melt” inside the body.

One of the main causes of the chemical deterioration of fats, oils and fatty foods during processing and storage is the **oxidation** of lipids. While the main trigger is oxygen, also other factors such as light and the presence of metals (that catalyze chain reactions initiated by free radicals) affect them. **Rancidity (or oxidation)** has unpleasant sensory properties (organoleptic) and can be toxic.

To understand why some oils become more oxidized or rancid than others, it is necessary to know that this process depends on the **natural antioxidants** they contain. Antioxidants -oxidation-inhibitors- are usually substances that can be extracted from the tissues of plants or animals. In plants, antioxidants prevent the oxidation of the vegetable cell, exposed to very high quantities of oxygen during photosynthesis.

The cell biological molecules are exposed to harmful atomic species called 'free radicals'. These free radicals - together with air pollution, smoke, herbicides and pesticides (which also generate free radicals) - affect hereditary DNA originating cell aging, appearance of certain cancers and cardiovascular diseases.

As free radicals are harmful to health, the body also requires antioxidants to catch them. That is why we need to ingest vitamin E as well as a variety of the many other antioxidants contained in vegetables of different colors, especially when polyunsaturated oils are consumed in large quantities. In this way, we prevent they become oxidized or rancid inside the body.

Unsaturated vegetable oils have attracted recent interest due to its composition and its associated phenolic antioxidant activity. Among phenols that stand out, hydroxytyrosol has been found in olive oils, resveratrol in dry fruit oils and sesamol in sesame seed oil.

It is still in research the role played by many of these bioactive phytochemicals on health. There is evidence that some compounds within the families of isoflavones, terpenoids, flavonoids and polyphenols may have a beneficial effect at different cellular levels, which are helpful in the prevention of pathologies such as degenerative diseases of the cardiovascular system and nervous system, as well as to halt processes related to carcinogenesis.

Oil extraction and its subsequent marketing

To choose the most appropriate oils for consumption is important to know what they contain and what methods are employed for their extraction and subsequent commercialization.

Extraction: To obtain the oil, it is necessary to break the vegetable cells by crushing, and then isolate it from other components of the cleaned seeds or fruits. The **triturating** is accomplished by rollers or millstones until a smooth paste is obtained which is submitted to a press where using mechanical devices pressure is applied to the paste squeezing out the oil. The **pressing or batter** of the dough can be made in cold or hot.

- **Cold Pressed**: the squeezed paste is carefully watched preventing that the pressure generated by the temperature may exceed 45 ° C - 113 ° F, to ensure the polyunsaturated fatty acids molecular stability

As a result of this process, the amount of oil extracted is smaller but the product is richer in unsaponifiable substances. This oil needs not to be refined, thus preventing the dissolution of waxes and other substances. These substances are formed by non fatty oil elements, such as phytosterols and vitamins. Some of these components are responsible for granting oils flavors akin to the fruit or seeds from which they come from, in addition to its medicinal properties.

The term "**first cold pressed**" was coined when the oil was obtained in pulp mills and a second pressing could be done adding hot water to the initial paste.

In many places, the extraction of cold-pressed oils is still carried out in a simple and traditional way. However, with the gradual emergence of new machinery, it is not being made a "**second cold pressing**." For this reason, this designation should be necessarily replaced by "**cold extraction**". This tendency is being increasingly observed in the labels.

- **Pressed or hot extraction**: the paste is heated before being squeezed. In this way you get more oil, but a significant amount of vitamins and phytosterols that are part of the oil are destroyed (antioxidants are burned).

- Extraction with solvents:

After applying pressure to the pulp, the residue still contains between 10% and 20% of oil. To exploit this residual oil the following processes are carried out:

Pressed pulp processing with solvents (ethylene dichloride hexane), which drag the waste oil.

By heating the residual oil, solvents evaporate and pure oil is obtained. Both, ethylene chloride as hexane are highly toxic, so it must be completely removed from the oil. In theory, the heating process does remove them, but in the practice, there can remain solvent residues. Besides, heat destroys vitamins and other active substances that may remain in the oil.

Refined Oils
The more you use pressure and heat for oil extraction, the more free fatty acids it contains, and refining it becomes necessary to remove them.

- **Refining** is a rather complex process intended to remove remove oil substances other than triglycerides (pure fat). The refining process consists of the following steps:

- Degumming

In this first phase, carbohydrates, proteins, resins and phospholipids (lecithin) industrially considered as impurities, are eliminated by using citric or phosphoric acid. Precisely in these oil "impurities" lie a good part of its medicinal properties. The sediment formed by all these substances is separated from oil by precipitation, and commercialized as lecithin.

- Neutralization

It aims to eliminate the free fatty acids responsible for the oil's acidity. This phase is accomplished by adding caustic soda, that forms soaps when becomes saponified with the free fatty acids, which are eliminated by centrifugation. This allows these oils to be heated at high temperatures without decomposing.

- Bleaching

It is achieved through the application of clay or carbon. This eliminates the carotenoids, minerals such as iron and copper, and other natural and beneficial substances contained in oil.

These complex processes of extraction and refining turn oil into an insipid **purified fatty substance** that tolerates frying and remains stable for a long time, but lacks the healthy natural benefits of virgin oils.

The most convenient oils for consumption

We can affirm that from the nutritional point of view, **the best oils are those cold extracted**. Both the pressed or hot extracted oil, as the refined one, reduce the content of substances that give the oil its taste, aroma, color and some of its most healthy components, like vitamins E and beta-carotene or provitamin A.

Fats

Butter

Butter is produced by churning milk cream. This action allows fat agglomeration in a single mass by breaking its surface tension, separating excess liquid that contains lactose, casein and other solids.

Through this process, patients with lactose intolerance or milk protein allergy may consume butter as a source of caloric fat.

Butter made from pasteurized milk is stable and can be kept refrigerated for a long period of time.

This milk by-product is a food **rich in saturated fat, cholesterol and calories**, recommendable for athletes or people with high energy consumption. Butter consumed with moderation is included in a healthy and balanced diet, except in special medical conditions (ex.: high blood cholesterol, atherosclerosis etc.). It is rich in vitamins A and D, and it is easy to digest. Geriatric and malnourished patients (with low blood cholesterol) can benefit from it.

It is not recommended frying with butter because of its low tolerance to heat.

TWO HIGH-QUALITY OILS

OLIVE OIL

Olive Oil: generic name for the oil that comes only from the olive tree fruit, excluding those obtained by using solvents, processes of re-esterification (reused), and blends with other oils. Nor does it apply to olive-pomace oils.

Virgin Olive Oils: are those obtained exclusively by physical processes and under certain temperature conditions which do not involve the alteration of the oil. It is a natural product that preserves the taste, aroma and vitamins of the fruit. It has the personality of the area where it comes from.

Classification of Olive Oils

1. **Organic extra virgin olive oil**. This oil should come from organically grown seeds (no agricultural chemicals) and be duly certified by authorized agencies. These seeds should be stored in silos equipped with aeration systems to optimize their preservation and freshness. This gourmet oil must be extracted using a traditional cold (reduced performance) procedure and must also have a packaging that protects them from light for their conservation. It is a high quality organic product that reaches consumer with a differential price.

2. **Extra virgin olive oil**. It is the pure olive juice obtained from mechanical pressing of olives harvested at the optimum time. It has a unique flavor and aroma, and has an acidity (free fatty acids) not exceeding 0.8 ° degrees. In addition to the organic extra virgin olive oil, this is highest quality and price olive oil in the market.

Extra virgin olive oils are free from any defect or chemical change and thus show a very interesting and pleasant range of aromas and flavors.

3. **Virgin or fine olive oil**: with an irreproachable taste and acidity of between 1° and 1.5°. Although inferior to extra, this oil is excellent for consuming.

   These are high quality olive oils but have not reached the maximum category for various reasons, and whose defects should be virtually imperceptible to the consumer. The grading (color, smell and taste) obtained by a trained tasting panel for virgin olive oil, should be equal or higher than 5.5 points.

4. **Refined olive oil**. It is obtained from virgin olive oils with high acidity, by using chemical processes. These oils have lost their organoleptic characteristics (color, smell and taste) and its natural properties. The acidity of this olive oil can not exceed 1.5°.

5. **Olive oil or pure olive oil**. This oil is **not** obtained by mechanical procedures, but comes from refining olive oil. Originally, these oils had a defect, so they have an added small amount of virgin olive oil in order to improve taste and reduce their acidity (not exceeding 1°). This is the traditionally consumed olive oil.

6. **"Lampante" – Lamp oil made of virgin olive oil**. This oil with an acidity exceeding 3° is not authorized for direct consumption. Its name comes from the utility that was given in the past as fuel for lamps or candles. It is used for refining because it is made from low quality olives (chopped olives, picked from the ground or from frost, etc.).

7. **Refined olive-pomace oil**. This type of oil is the result of chemically refined marc (bones and remains of olive once oil is extracted) by pressing of olives. The vegetable fat obtained is mixed with a determined proportion of a virgin olive oil (other than lampante).

Characteristics of Extra Virgin Olive Oils

Acidity: The rules issued by the **International Olive Council** set a maximum acidity of 0.8 °% for Virgin-Extra or Extra-Virgin olive oil. This limit is considered very realistic, since most of extra virgin oils are commercialized with a total acidity of between 0.3 ° and 0.8 °.

Acidity is one of the chemical parameters for olive oils, and indicates the amount of free fatty acid oil contained in the oil (expressed as% oleic acid). A low acidity in oils is a guarantee that **virgin oils** were produced from healthy olives and in the best conditions during all phases of the process. That is why each category of virgin olive oils must have a certain degree of acidity.

However, experts virgin olive tasters celebrate that finally it has been obviated the mandatory mention (in the label) of the acidity degree, which created confusion in the majority of consumers that were comparing the **acidity** of **extra virgin olive oil** with **olive oil** (mixed refined and virgin). This confusion, which still persists, is because **olive oil** can be made to have higher or lesser degree of acidity depending on the proportion of refined olive oil mixed with **extra virgin oil** as determined by the producer.
It is necessary to consider that olive oil quality arises in the fields, from a combination of environmental factors (climate and soil), genetic (olive variety) and agronomic (cultivation techniques) as well as the processes carried out from harvesting to bottling. This feature is known as:

Protected Designation of Origin, whose acronym (PDO) classifies oils obtained through olives from a specific geographic area. This olive oil has to be produced and bottled in the designed area, besides being subjected to different types of controls to ensure its origin.

Extra virgin olive oils tasting: oils that present a clean look after filtration and decantation are valued as good or normal. Those which are cloudy, dirty or dark are considered defective.

The normal range of colors includes the following shades: straw yellow, golden yellow, yellow-green, green and deep green. Oils are considered defective when presenting atypical and unusual colors: red, white, brown or blackish, muddy and dark.

As for flavors, the golden-yellow shades usually correspond to fresh olive oils, extracted from ripe olives of late harvest. The yellow-green tones are unique to fruity olive oil (with just a point of pleasant bitter) resulting from the unripened fruits.

The valuation of aromatic and taste sensations can be "pleasant and unpleasant."

- Pleasant: aromas and flavors of ripe fruit, unripe fruit, olive fruit, apple, green leaves or grass.
- Unpleasant: aromas and tastes vinegary, winy, tart, spicy or intense bitter, wet or moldy, overheated, to frost olives, metallic, slops or rotten, fusty or poorly stored and rancid olives.

Modern production of olive oil

In most modern plants for extra virgin olive oil production, clean fruits are carefully crushed in cold, in a two phase's mill until a paste is obtained. Then this paste is kneaded in a stainless steel blade mixer with electronic temperature control set to operate at less than 73.4 ° F - 23 ° C (the lower the temperature, the better the quality of the product).

The homogenized pulp to 73.4 ° F - 23 ° C passes from the mixer to the horizontal centrifuge for decanting. The purpose here is to separate the oil from 99% of the remaining components; in this case, from the crushed olive. The remaining one percent is separated by vertical centrifugation, finishing the process the same day of recollection. The product is accomplished **without crimping**, by "**cold extraction**", producing an extra virgin oil of high quality.

World production and consumption of olive oil

Olive oil production has been always associated with countries in the Mediterranean region: **Spain, Italy, Greece, Portugal, Turkey, Tunisia and Morocco**. These seven countries account for 90% of world production.

Other countries like Australia and the United States are starting to increase their olive oil production. China also has a significant number of olive trees and is starting its production of extra virgin olive oils.

The major consuming countries are also the major producing countries. The European Union countries account for 71% of global consumption. The Mediterranean countries account for 77% of global consumption. Other consuming countries are the United States, Canada, Australia and Japan.

AVOCADO OIL

The avocado, known in South America as aguacate, is a pre-Columbian crop widely spread from Mexico to the north of Chile. Later, Europeans imported the avocado and made it one of their favorite fruits, ascribing it aphrodisiac properties and incorporating it to their diet.

The extra virgin avocado oil has virtues that make it a high quality product. It has a very similar chemical composition to olive oil, however, although it contains higher levels of vitamin E, beta-sitosterol -*reducer of blood cholesterol levels*- and chlorophyll, compared to extra virgin olive oil sample, it shows lower levels of squalene - *key in the synthesis of cholesterol*- and polyphenols, *antioxidant micronutrients*. Chlorophyll is a pigment that is present in plants and green algae, and is responsible for light energy absorption in the photosynthesis process.

Although chlorophyll may adversely affect the oil's oxidizing stability producing photo-oxidation, consumers value their green color as a desired attribute. To increase the oil's oxidizing stability during its useful life, exposure of the product to light must be avoided by using dark-glass bottles. Likewise, the contact of the liquid with the oxygen must be prevented by using nitrogen in storage tanks and during the packaging process.

The world production of extra virgin avocado oil (for cooking purposes) has been recently increased. However, it has rapidly been established as a gourmet basis for the Mediterranean diet.

Since 1999, New Zealand is the world's largest producer of extra virgin avocado oil. However, in the last years Chile has developed this gourmet cooking oil and its world sale has greatly increased.

Experts consider extra virgin avocado oil will have a future as promising as olive oil.

Action of heat on extra virgin olive and avocado oils

Under the right conditions of temperature, without reaching the smoking point, the olive and avocado extra virgin oils show no substantial change in their structure and retain their original properties better than other healthy oils. This is due to its small content of polyunsaturated fatty acids and its higher proportion of monounsaturated fatty acids (oleic acid).

This feature makes them the cold-pressed vegetable oils with greater stability to heat, unlike virgin oils derived from seeds that contain polyunsaturated fatty acids, which are easily altered by heat.

The recipes in this book that include techniques for heating oil have been elaborated exclusively with olive or avocado extra virgin oil.

FOOD GROUPS AND PORTIONS SIZE

The food pyramid shown below has been modified to present a new hierarchy of foods that endows a greater value to the intake of vegetables, fruits, unsaturated oils, and white meat.

Food Pyramid of the Mediterranean Diet
Modified for Weight Loss by Dr. Durand

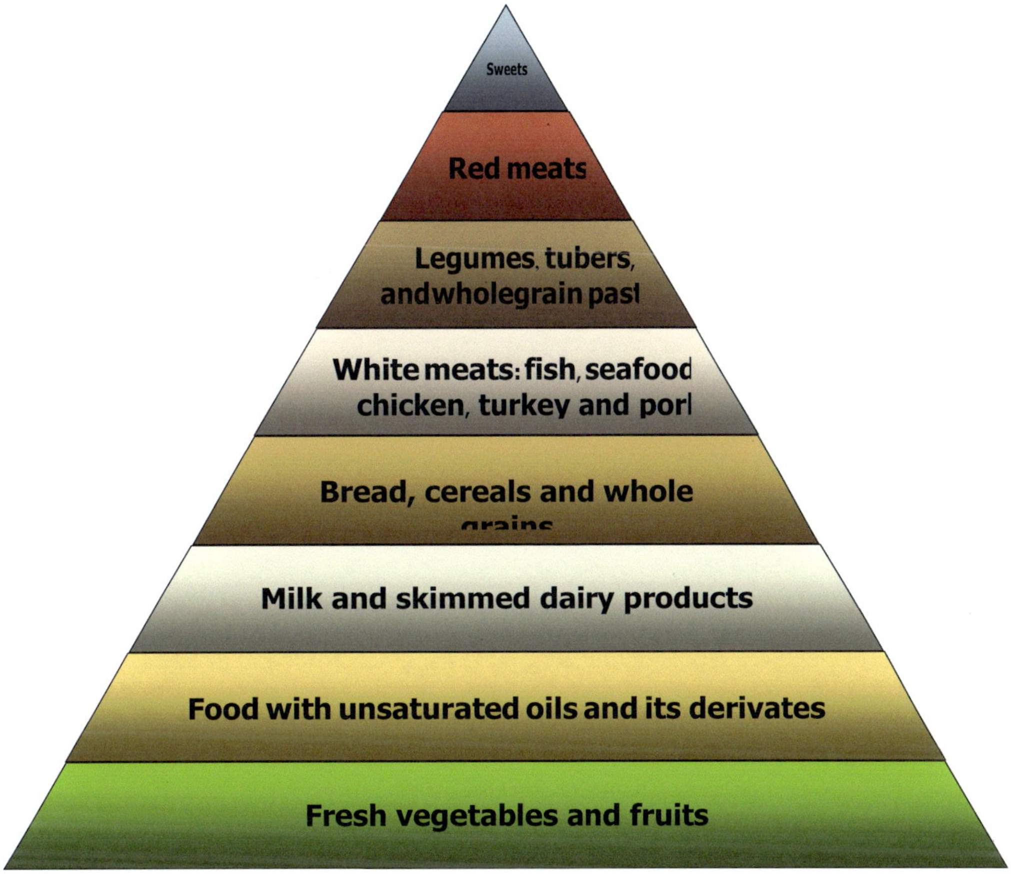

1. Fresh vegetables and fruits
2. Foods containing unsaturated oils and derivatives:
   extra virgin oils, dried fruits, seeds, olives and avocado
   (consume in moderation because of their high calorie content)
3. Milk and skimmed dairy products, eggs (ideally with high levels of omega-3)
4. Bread, cereals, whole grains and dehydrated fruits
   (consume in moderation because of their high calorie content)
5. White meats: fish, seafood, chicken, turkey and pork
6. Legumes, tubers and whole grain pasta
7. Red meats
8. Sweets

Portions Size

Food portions ingested in adequate amounts should be sized to improve nutrition and to expand the food groups that we should consume.

It is possible to achieve a balance between caloric intake and expenditure if eating habits are improved and physical activity is practiced regularly.

However, it is also important to know that the body's biological efficiency is large. For that reason, to achieve weight loss it is more important to reduce calorie intake than to do exercise.

Parents should become models for their children, inculcating in them a healthy lifestyle based on a balanced caloric intake, in choosing appropriate food and eating in moderation.

Detailed Food information

1. Fresh vegetables and fruits:

Four color vegetables:
We recommend eating daily at least 2 to 4 different color vegetables from the following options:
1 cup varied cooked vegetables
1 cup varied cooked vegetables, juiced
1 cup varied raw vegetable salad
1 cup varied raw vegetables, juiced
2 cups raw green vegetables

Four colors fruits:
We recommend eating daily 2 to 4 servings of different color fruits options:

1 medium fruit
1 cup chopped fruit
1/2 cup fruit juice

Why choose fresh fruits and vegetables?

- Because carbohydrates from vegetables and fruits are easy to digest and provide energy without getting you fat.
- Because fiber, a significant component of vegetables and fruits, regulates the absorption of nutrients by acting as a mesh, gradually releasing substances that the body needs to incorporate. Furthermore, is responsible for retaining harmful substances such as cholesterol or excess fat.

Fiber increases the volume of the bolus, which gives a greater feeling of satiety, stimulates intestinal movement and facilitates feces elimination.

In some cases it is recommended to replace fruit-juice, adequately portioned, by whole fruit, preferably with skin. It should be mentioned that the addition of raw foods to diet can lead to food adaptation problems. Intestinal flora lives on what we eat: changes in the diet may produce flatulence and digestive discomfort for several days. This is so because some intestinal flora bacteria disappear, while other bacteria repopulate the intestinal mucosa.

It is recommended, wherever possible, to purchase and consume fresh foods. However, instead of eating any fast food, it is preferable to take home some frozen or canned vegetables and/or fruits.

To choose canned or frozen foods precautions should be taken into account as suggested below:

Vegetables: choose those packaged in water or having low sodium. Wash vegetables several times with fresh water before eating it to remove the extra salt that was added for preservation. Do not choose vegetables that have added butter, cream or cheese.

Fruits: select low-calorie products. However if you choose caned fruits prefer those canned in 100% of its juice. These contain less sugar than those packed in syrup. To discard added sugar, the fruit should be washed several times with fresh water before use.

Almost all canned or frozen fruits and vegetables have been processed immediately after being harvested, which prevents the loss of many of their nutrients.

2. Unsaturated oils and their derivatives

Foods containing unsaturated oils and their derivatives (be aware these food have lots of calories).

- extra virgin oils
- dry fruits
- seeds
- olives
- avocado

We recommend eating 2 to 4 daily portions of any of the following options:

1 tablespoon extra virgin olive oil
3 to 5 olives
¼ medium avocado
3 to 4 dry fruits
1 tablespoon seeds

Why is it important to consume fat?

Because fat is a source of energy. In addition, carries fat-soluble vitamins A, D, E and K, which need an oily substrate (animal or vegetal) to be absorbed by the body.

Bile and pancreatic enzymes are required to digest fat. Bile's lecithin (and bile salts), act as a *detergent or cleaner*, allowing fat (oil) and water to get mixed. These detergents inhibit the formation of an interface between water and oil. This happens because one end of the lecithin molecule (and bile salts) is soluble in water while the other end is soluble in oil.

Why we prefer vegetable oils to animal oils?

Animal oils (fats) are saturated and contain cholesterol. Instead, vegetable oils have no cholesterol and contain unsaturated fatty acids. Some vegetables derived oils contain large amounts of essential oils. However, some have saturated fatty acids too.

Essential polyunsaturated fats, also known as omega 3 and omega 6, are not produced by the body and are acquired only from food. Some sources of these essential fats include extra virgin oils obtained from seeds, fruits, nuts, legumes and cereals.

Medical Note: Another excellent source of essential fats is fish, which has been included in the modified food pyramid within the group of white meat.

Extra virgin oils

Extra virgin oils are vegetable oils primarily for culinary use, which are extracted from fruits or seeds.

Dry fruits

These are foods distinguished by their high energetic and caloric delivery. They should be present in all diets. Their contribution is invaluable in the kitchen, adding different flavors to simple foods.

Dry fruits fall into two main groups:

In the first group are those that have hard shell, such as **almonds**, **cashews nuts**, **hazelnuts**, **macadamias**, **peanuts, walnuts**, **Brazil nuts**, **pecans**, **pine nuts**, **pistachios**, **sunflower seeds** and **sesame seeds**, among the most common. These nuts are poor in water and rich in fat, so their consumption should be moderated.

In the second group are dried or desiccated fruits, which have been included within the group of carbohydrates rich food sources in the modified food pyramid of our book.

Almonds
They are an important source of protein and minerals such as calcium, magnesium, potassium, copper, phosphorus and zinc. Almonds have large amounts of monounsaturated fatty acids, contains vitamin E and, to a lesser extent, vitamin B 6. It is also the nut with more fiber in its composition.

Cashew nuts
This fruit contains a high proportion of monounsaturated fatty acids, folic acid, vitamins B1, B2, magnesium, calcium and potassium, which benefit the nervous system.

Hazelnuts
They represent one of the oldest food crops. They are high in monounsaturated and polyunsaturated fats. Hazelnuts also provide minerals such as copper, magnesium, calcium, potassium and phosphorus. They are a good natural source of vitamin E, and B vitamins such as B6 and folic acid.

Macadamias
Macadamia nut or Australian nut is the youngest among dry fruits. It contains a high proportion of monounsaturated fats, is rich in fiber, calcium, phosphorus, iron and vitamin B1.

Peanuts
Peanuts seeds are high in protein and rich in antioxidants. Eating large amounts of peanut butter is a habit ingrained since childhood at many households in the United States of America. However, being a high-calorie food, it is necessary to monitor intake to avoid overweight or obesity, both in children and adults.

The peanut contains a high proportion of monounsaturated fat. However, during it's processing to peanut butter it can be modified to trans oil, which is a more solid fat that has a tendency to aggregate, stick and deposit in cells, organs and arteries, causing health problems. It is important to mention that eating peanuts and its derivatives may cause allergic reactions in some people.

Walnuts
The fruit of the Walnut tree contains seed with significant amounts of polyunsaturated fatty acids (omega 3 and omega 6). In addition, this nut provides vitamins E, B1 and B6, fiber and minerals such as copper, zinc, potassium, magnesium, calcium and phosphorus.

Brazil nuts
It is the fruit of a wild tree that grows in the Amazon jungle, also known as coquito of Brazil. This nut is found inside a large shell and stands out by its high concentration of minerals such as calcium, iron and zinc. Thanks to the Amazon soil, where it grows, it is rich in selenium and has powerful antioxidants. It provides monounsaturated and polyunsaturated fat in equal proportions, as well as fiber and vitamins, such as folic acid, calcium, etc.

Pecans
Pecans are rich in monounsaturated fatty acids and provide moderate amounts of protein, fiber and sterols. They furnish folic acid and minerals like magnesium, calcium, potassium and phosphorus.

Pine nuts
From the culinary point of view, pine nuts are fruits, but in the botanical sense they are seeds. They provide vitamins B1 and are rich in minerals such as potassium, phosphorus, magnesium, iron, folic acid and calcium. Pine nuts are high in unsaturated fat, predominantly polyunsaturated.

Pistachios
This fruit contains an elongated and edible seed. After almond, it is the dry fruit with more protein. The pistachio is high in monounsaturated fat. It also provides vitamins such as E and appreciable amounts of copper, magnesium, phosphorus and calcium.

Seeds

Sunflower seeds
Sunflower seeds are rich in minerals such as phosphorus, magnesium and potassium. It also contains polyunsaturated fatty acids and provides significant amounts of calcium and vitamin E.

Sesame seeds
The sesame is a plant grown for its seeds. These are rich in protein and have high levels of unsaturated fats. They are source of different minerals such as calcium, iron and zinc, and provide B group vitamins and vitamin E. Sesame seeds also have significant amounts of fiber, so that their consumption is beneficial for regulating bowel function.

Culinary Note: in order to conserve dried fruit for a longer time, we recommend storing it in an airtight container, for up to 6 months in the refrigerator and for 1 year in the freezer.

Olives

Purchase green or black olives packed in glass jars. Prefer only those that are packed in brine (salt water), avoiding any type of vinegar marinated olives, aromatic herbs, spices, etc.

Packaged olives stored at room temperature in its original container, are preserved for about 1 year.

After opening the original package, refrigerate them in salted water inside a glass jar.

Avocado

This fruit (also considered a vegetable) contains a high percentage of monounsaturated and polyunsaturated fats. It is the fruit with antioxidant properties par excellence. This is due to its high content of vitamins, especially E. It is also rich in proteins and minerals.

It is called "vegetable butter" because of the creamy texture of the mature pulp and its high caloric value. We recommend consuming it in moderation.

3. Nonfat dairy products and eggs (omega-3)

We recommend eating 2 to 4 portions daily of any of the following options:

½ cup skim milk
½ cup nonfat yogurt or kefir
½ cup low-fat cottage cheese
¼ cup low-fat feta cheese
¼ cup low fat ricotta cheese
¼ cup low-fat mozzarella cheese
1 to 2 eggs omega 3 (consume less than one yolk per day)

Milk

Milk is a product that contains a great variety of nutrients, both energetic (fat and carbohydrates) and structural (proteins).

Why we include dairy products?
Dairy products are the most calcium-rich foods. They have the additional advantage that calcium derived from milk is well absorbed because of the presence of lactose, vitamin D, and the adequate calcium / phosphorus proportion. In general, they are a good source of vitamins, especially retinol and riboflavin.

Lactose intolerance: is the gastrointestinal distress caused by the decreased level of intestinal lactase. Lactase is an enzyme found in the intestinal mucosa necessary for the proper degradation of lactose (milk sugar) into glucose and galactose. In some individuals, especially the old, the low levels of this enzyme in the intestine prevents the metabolism of lactose remaining itself in the gut producing an osmotic event that results in abdominal pain, bloating and diarrhea. Lactase levels are also genetically determined in the individual.

Mi**lk allergy** is an immune reaction to milk proteins, especially casein and its peptides.

The milk proteins are classified into two groups: casein (80%) and serum proteins (20%). There is a close relationship between the amount of fat and the amount of protein in milk: The higher the amount of fat, the more protein.

Other considerations: casein begins its digestion in the stomach by the action of renin and pepsin, gastric enzymes whose secretion decrease with age, becoming insufficient in many cases. Moreover, milk neutralizes gastric acidity, making it more difficult for the elderly to digest it.

Modified milk: a very important aspect of our eating habits is the increasing use of low-calorie products, among them milk and skim milk. The main difference between whole milk (3.7% fat), semi skimmed (between 1.5 and 2% fat) and skim (less than 1% fat) is its fat content, cholesterol, and fat soluble vitamins (A and D). Skim milk is a low-calorie food that has one of the highest nutrient concentrations. Its consumption can be very useful for people that suffer abnormal fat levels in blood, high cholesterol, overweight or obesity.

Yogurt: is the best-known fermented milk product. It is obtained by adding a microbial culture to milk, fostering its coagulation by a decrease in the pH. These microorganisms, *Streptococcus thermophilus*, *Lactobacillus bulgaricus*, *Streptococcus lactis*, *Lactobacillus acidophylus*, *Lactobacillus casei Shirota* and *inmunitans,* cause a partial conversion of lactose into lactic acid, which protects the intestinal flora. It is easily digested because it is converted by the action of bacteria (yogurt) in protein fragments (peptides) and amino acids, thereby facilitating their digestion and absorption, thus facilitating its absorption. Calcium is in the form of calcium lactate, which is digested and assimilated better. The nutritional value of yogurt is almost identical to that of milk from which it derived, keeping the regenerative and restorative properties of the intestinal flora in balance. Its storage time is greater than that of fresh milk.

Kefir: it comes from the Caucasus Mountains region, where it was cultivated for centuries and then spread throughout the world. As food, kefir is a probiotic drink that has undergone a triple fermentation: lactic, alcoholic and gaseous. The kefir granules consist of 9 bacteria that depending on the culture incubation temperatures, transform lactose into lactic acid, produce CO2 (gas) and then ethanol. The kefir regenerates the intestinal flora, has an antiseptic function and cleanses the body of pathogenic bacteria, which are neutralized by the beneficial ones.

Cheese

According to the dictionary definition of the Royal Spanish Academy, cheese is "the product obtained by curd maturation, having special characteristics for each type according to their origin or manufactured method".

Cheese is obtained as follows: milk and vinegar are mixed so that milk casein flocculates (procedure to precipitate or flocculate the dissolved substances) forming clots or "curds" used to prepare the cheese, while on the surface serum remains still containing many nutrients.

This process, especially in aged cheeses, results in a product where lactose disappears, and proteins and fats are hydrolyzed, thus enabling its use in most people with lactose intolerance and/or allergy to casein.

Classification according to its processing procedure:

Fresh cheeses are those in which the elaboration only consists of pasteurization, coagulation, and draining of the serum, without going through a maturation process.

Mature, **cured** or **blue cheeses** are those that acquire different aromas, flavors and textures through maturation techniques.

Melted cheeses are made from one or various cheeses mixed under heat. Then other ingredients such as milk powder, whey, cream or butter, water and salt are added.

Medical Note: due to its high caloric content, mature or melted cheese should be eaten in moderation.

Why we recommend young cheese?
Because during its preparation, more fat has been extracted from the "fresh" or young cheese than from the mature, cured or blue cheese. Fresh cheese nutrients are better assimilated than those produced by fermentation using lactic acid bacteria or rennet. It is noteworthy that although fresh cheese has less calcium than mature or concentrated cheeses, it is better assimilated. This is because it contains less saturated fat, but mainly due to its greater richness in lactose. This, by encouraging the formation of lactic acid, stimulates digestive activity, and consequently, the absorption of many other nutrients, especially calcium. Fresh cheeses are characterized for their mild flavor and soft texture.

Fresh cheese, despite all its benefits and its high nutritional value, also supplies a certain amount of saturated fat and cholesterol, so its consumption should be in moderation and accompanied with vegetable products rich in fiber, to modulate saturated fat absorption.

Some of the most popular fresh-soft cheeses

Cottage Cheese: very popular in the United States. It is a product with a soft, moist, granular and creamy texture. It is elaborated with semi skimmed or skim milk.

Its fat content is 3% and in its lighter versions has less than 2%. It is a food rich in protein, calcium, vitamin B12, zinc and folic acid.

Feta Cheese: is a traditional product of Greece, Turkey and Bulgaria. It is elaborated with sheep, goat or cow milk. It's saltier than other fresh cheeses (**should be avoided by hypertensive patients**) and has no outer crust. It has a natural white color and a soft and flexible consistency.

Its lactic fat content is 43%. In the traditional feta cheese elaboration it is not allowed to use preservatives.

Fresh Mozzarella Cheese: is known worldwide as the pizza's base. It is elaborated from cows or buffaloes milk. The mozzarella cheese has a soft and elastic texture - (pasta filata) – and has a mild flavor and aroma. In some areas of southern Italy, it is consumed within hours of its preparation.

Ricotta Cheese: it is a cheese made originally in Italy that has a moist, soft or granular texture. It is prepared with milk whey or cheese whey adding milk curd generated by heat, lactic acid bacteria and organic acids. The resulting characteristics of ricotta cheese depend on the particular type of coagulant used.

It contains more lactose than other fresh cheeses, so it can cause gas, bloating, cramps, diarrhea and other digestive problems in people with lactose intolerance.

Eggs

The **egg white** represents 60% of egg weight. It is a viscous and transparent substance, and coagulates at 150 º F - 65 º C, taking on a white-color. It contains 90% of water and 10% of high biological value protein.

The **yolk** or vitelo is about 30% of the complete egg. Contains 30% fat, 15% protein, 45% water, minerals (calcium, phosphorus, iron), fat soluble vitamins (A, D, E) and soluble (B1, B2). Its different fatty acids proportions largely depend on the bird feeding. An egg contains about 7.5 g total lipids, of which 2.0 g are saturated, 1.1 g polyunsaturated fatty acids and 3.0 g monounsaturated fatty acids. The yolk color varies depending on the amount of pigments that are added to the bird feed, which does not affect its nutritional quality. The yolk is high in cholesterol.

Important Note: **omega-3 eggs** come from birds that have been fed with flaxseeds rich in omega 3, vitamin E (antioxidant), natural grass and concentrates of corn.

How to select and store eggs

Fresh eggs are recognized by their bright waxy skin, which eventually becomes opaque. When fresh, the eggs have pleasant smell and taste; chilled, stay fresh for up to 28 days.

4. Breads, cereals and grains, and dried fruits

We recommend eating 1 to 2 portions daily of any of the following options:

1 slice wholegrain bread
½ cup wholegrain cereal
½ cup brown rice
2 to 3 medium or large dry fruits
3 to 5 small dried fruit

Bread

Bread is a food product made from baking flour mixed with water or milk and then baked adding other ingredients. The most appropriate for consumption is the wholegrain bread, elaborated with grains that have not been refined.

Cereals and whole grains

Why is it important to consume them?

Cereals and **whole grains** are **carbohydrates** rich seeds that keep their outer-shell and the germ. They are **rich in fiber**, B vitamins, minerals and vegetable protein. Fiber has the ability to enhance peristalsis without being digested by the body, slowing down digestion.

The slower the digestion and absorption of its carbohydrates, the slower will be the absorption of sugar and the release of insulin. This avoids the sudden changes in blood glucose and fat accumulation in adipose tissue cells.

Glycemic index (GI): is a measure of the effect caused on blood glucose by carbohydrates ingested through food.

Foods with low glycemic index contain complex sugars that are slowly digested and absorbed, producing a lower blood glucose level.

Refined carbohydrates (white sugar) have a high glycemic index, which reflects the rapid absorption of glucose into the blood. The glucose rapidly releases insulin from the pancreas, which lowers blood sugar levels. Glucose is introduced into the adipose cells, which convert glucose into fat for storage. We should add **fiber** to our diet to reduce the negative effect of high glycemic index foods.

Dried Fruits

They have been included in the high carbohydrate group of foods because they contain large amounts of simple carbohydrates and fiber. Due to their high sugar content, their consumption should be moderated or restricted (especially in diabetic patients).

Dried fruit such as prunes, apricots, dried apricots, plums, dried figs, raisins, etc., and dates * are part of the traditional cuisine of many countries and are also a suitable complement to our diet. They share the high caloric index with hard-shelled nuts, but its nutritional composition is different.

The drying or dehydration process is intended to reduce the water content in the fruit in order to inhibit the activity of germs that need moisture to live. This preservation process increases the concentration of nutrients (simple carbohydrates and sugars), adding "caloric density" to the fruit.

Their soluble fiber content gives them a laxative property. They are a good source of potassium, calcium and iron.

* Dates are different from other dried fruits as they are let to dry still hanging from the tree and are collected only once dried. In contrast, other fruits are harvested first and dried later on.

5. White meat: fish, seafood, chicken, turkey and pork

We recommend eating 1 to 2 portions daily, alternating protein sources eating the following portions:

¾ to 1 cup (125 gr. - 4.3 oz.) of fat-free white meat
such as fish or shellfish (up to 2 times per week),
poultry or pork.

In nutritional terms, the fundamental difference between red and white meat consists in the amount and quality of fat they contain. White meats are those with less fat and, generally, are of better quality.

The **Fruits of the Sea** are living aquatic animals, usually fish, but they can also be mollusks, crustaceans and cephalopods (shellfish) or even marine mammals.

Beneficial omega-3 derivates

Overall, there are two essential fatty acids whose oil derivates have biological antagonistic effects in man: the omega-6 or linoleic acid (pro-inflammatory polyunsaturated oil), and the omega-3 or linolenic acid (pro-anti-inflammatory polyunsaturated oil).

Omega-3 polyunsaturated oils are those animal or vegetable oils derived from the essential linolenic acid oil which is essential because it can not be produced by the human body and must be obtained through food. The omega-3 oils derivates EPA and DHA are the truly beneficial derivates of linolenic acid. The human body can produce them in small amounts. However, they are critical for neurological integrity as well as other essential biologic functions.

In nature, EPA and DHA are produced by polar seas microalgae, which are later eaten by fish. This is why only oils derived from marine animals contain the beneficial derivates of omega-3 oils (DHA and EPA).

We normally keep a healthy balance in the consumption of omega-6 and omega-3 oils. However, it is suggested we should eat a little bit more omega-3 than omega-6 oils. This would allow the body to produce more EPA and DHA omega-3 derivates than omega-6 derivate oils.

In order to consume food or commercial oils that provide significant amounts of EPA and DHA directly, it is necessary to know the source (generally marine) of these oils. They have to be from an animal source as these linolenic acid derivates are produced by marine polar phytoplankton and are retained by animals that feed on them.

In the animal kingdom, significant amounts of the linolenic acid (omega-3) derivates EPA and DHA can only be found in fish. Omega-3 oils derivates can also be found in specially fed mammals or birds supplemented with foods containing significant amounts of marine feed or algae that have a high concentration of linolenic acid (and their beneficial derivates). Thus, some mammals or birds can produce meat or eggs with high levels of omega-3 oils having also higher levels of EPA and DHA too. For example, in the market there are eggs and other products with larger amounts of omega-3 oil (and its derivatives) than the usual farmed raised eggs.

In the vegetal kingdom, omega-3 oils (but not their beneficial derivates) are present in oils from flaxseed, soybeans, wheat germ and nuts. Omega-6 oils are present in oils from sunflower, corn, soybeans and cotton. No EPA or DHA is found in vegetable oils.

There are companies that use transgenic fungus to produce EPA and DHA from linolenic acid. This creates a non-marine biological source to produce the beneficial linolenic acid derivatives and may have the advantage of not containing mercury, now-a-days a known contaminate of marine origin oils.

In conclusion, eating vegetable oil that contains omega-3 oils does not provide the same beneficial effects of consuming marine origin oils, as they do not provide the derivatives EPA and DHA that are truly the beneficial oils.

Medical Note: to obtain the pharmacologic benefit of EPA and DHA, the fatty acids omega-3 derivates can also be consumed directly from fish oil capsules (or liquid tonics) that contain them. These high quality products are sold commercially.

Fish

Proteins: As with meat from ruminants and poultry, proteins found in fish contain all essential amino acids.

Fat: Fish is appreciated according to its fat content and are classified into three groups:

Lean or white fishes live in the deep sea and make limited journeys, so they do not need to accumulate fat. Most lean fish have white flesh. Depending on the species, they contain from 1% to 2% fat, which they store mainly in the liver. They are easy to digest. This group includes: monkfish, catfish, sole, grouper, cod, and hake, among others.

In the United States of America, the farm-raised white meat tilapia is the third most consumed aquatic product after shrimp and salmon.

Semi fatty fishes live in mid-depths and their journeys are usually long. They have a fat content intermediate between lean and blue fish, ranging from 2% to 7%. They are less digestible and provide more calories than lean fish. The best known include: cod, conger eel, sturgeon, trout, black grouper, yellow perch, bass, and sea bream.

Oily or Blue fishes make long journeys, so they need to accumulate fat in their muscles. Oily fishes contain between 8 to 15% of fat, mostly distributed in their tissues. The amount of fat influences their coloration, thus most of oily fish are blue.

The fish in cold waters has fatty streaks much thicker than the fish obtained by fish farming. It is important to mention that in the commercialization of fatty fish, unlike white or red meat, they are quoted by their fat content. Fat is seen between the muscle fibers, especially in the tuna and salmon.

Among the oily fish are the following: anchovy, herring, salmon, tuna, albacore, white tuna, sea bream, white anchovy, mackerel, sardine and swordfish.

Important Note: this classification is not well defined because the fat content in some fish varies throughout the year and is intrinsically dependent on several factors.

These factors can be:
- The age and size of fish: at more age and weight, the higher the proportion of fat.
- The fishing season: some species accumulate more fat in certain seasons; for example, mackerel contains twice as much omega 3 in autumn than in winter.
- The environment in which they live: marine fish contain more omega 3 than freshwater fish.
- Water temperature: cold water fish like salmon and mackerel, are more nutrient-rich.
- Feeding of fish: those that feed on plankton, rich in omega 3, such as anchovies, tuna, salmon or mackerel, have higher amounts of this fatty acid.

- The distance covered before spawning: fish accumulate fat as energy reserves prior to reproduction, and the king salmon, unlike the pink salmon, has large deposits of fat because it travels longer distances before spawning.

Medical Note: methyl mercury is a metal that can be found in some fish, mainly in the largest ones.

The **fat** of fish, especially of oily fish, is rich in polyunsaturated fatty acids omega-3 (linolenic acid) as well as their beneficial derivates (DHA and EPA). These derivates have antithrombotic, anti-inflammatory, anti-arrhythmic and anti-atherogenic agents, which prevent arteriosclerosis, heart attack and cancer.

Important note: buy the fish or shellfish at the end of your food purchases. The macerated or marinated fish should be kept in the refrigerator, never at room temperature.

The fish should have bright eyes and the skin color should be well defined and even. The gills should be intensely red, the fin stiff, and the scales shining. The flesh should be firm to touch, if it cedes to your finger pressure, this indicates that product is not fresh. It should smell like the sea, never like ammonia.

Food poisoning from eating fish:

Ciguatera poisoning: this can happen when eating a reef fish (any fish living in warm tropical waters) that has eaten some poisonous food. This toxin does not disappear when the fish is cooked or frozen.

Scombroid poisoning: This occurs when eating fish that is not fresh or has been mishandled, as it accumulates large amounts of histamine and histidine. When fish spoils, histidine (an amino acid) degrades to histamine, a substance responsible for allergic reactions signs and symptoms. Fish can be frozen for up to 6 months.

Medical Note: patients with chronic liver diseases, the immune suppressed (cancer, diabetes, AIDS, etc.), and women whose ovaries have been surgically removed should not eat fresh seafood (especially oysters) because of the risk of contamination with the bacterium *Vibrio vulnificus*. In general, these patients are advised to cook their seafood.

Seafood

Shellfish more frequently consumed fall into two classes: mollusks and crustaceans.

Mollusks: oysters, squid, octopus, mussels, scallops, clams, mussels, oysters, sea snail, etc., are low in calories and saturated fat. They are an excellent source of iron, besides being rich in protein. They contain iodine, sodium, potassium, phosphorus, copper, cobalt, magnesium and to a lesser amount fluoride. They also provide B vitamins (B1, B2, B6 and B12), vitamin A, and significant amounts of calcium, trace elements and fatty acids, like omega 3.

Crustaceans: lobsters, shrimps, crabs, king prawn and goose barnacle; share their nutritional qualities with mollusks. Crustaceans have less fat than seafood but they provide substantial levels of cholesterol.

Characteristics and storage of fresh seafood:

- It is important that the eyes and the antennae of live crustaceans (lobsters, shrimp, and crab) are bright and erect, and that they also can move their legs.
- Mollusks sold alive should keep their two shells closed. All fresh mollusks should have no cracks in their shells, neither ammonia odor.

Take them home in containers with ice, and refrigerate immediately to avoid risk of poisoning.

If you are not going to consume them in 24 hours, it is best to freeze them. They hold up to 6 months. Avoid eating them raw. Discard any shellfish that keep their shells closed after cooking.

Medical Note: the patients with hepatic impairment should not eat shellfish (oysters).

Frozen seafood: Now-a-days, the food industry offers a variety of frozen or canned products of the highest quality.

The potential risks of eating fish, mollusks and crustaceans are avoided buying them at recognized distribution centers, properly labeled, subjected to a proper handling, preparation and preservation.

We recommend choosing foods packed in water. To discard the salt they contain, it is convenient to wash the product several times with fresh water before use.

Chicken

Chicken meat, **especially breast meat**, is rich in protein and is one of the meats that have less fat. It stands out for its high content of vitamin B3 and folic acid; also has iron, zinc, phosphorus and potassium.

Turkey

Turkey meat, **especially breast meat**, is easy to digest. Has low fat and low cholesterol, being the thigh meat the leanest. It has the same biologic protein value as in other meats, is rich in potassium, magnesium and vitamin B 3 or niacin.

As in chicken, most of its fat content is underneath the skin, making it easy to remove. The turkey breast contains little fat.

One of the biggest advantages of chicken or turkey is that their consumption may be appropriate in hypoallergenic diets, and are ideal for regimes low in saturated fat and cholesterol.

Pork

Pork (**loin or defatted chop**) is a healthy option in a balanced diet because it contains high quality protein. It also has minerals, especially organic iron molecules, which stimulates the absorption of mineral iron that is essential to prevent iron deficiency anemia.

It also contains zinc, phosphorus, sodium and potassium as well as vitamins C. Except for its low folic acid content, it has from 8 to 10 times more thiamine or vitamin B1 than other meats and is a good source of vitamin B 12.

Characteristics of fresh white meat:

Usually, meat is fresh if its consistency is firm, maintains its polish when cut and presents a pleasant color and odor.

While being sold, fresh meat should always be kept in refrigerated containers protected from public contact. The pieces, cuts and animal categories must be differentiated.

Conservation of fresh white meat:

The meat will be preserved in the refrigerator up to 3 to 4 days, however once chopped or grounded, no more than 2 days. Always wrap the meat with plastic film (plastic wrap), aluminum foil or store it in an airtight container. Meat should be cleaned with a damp cloth instead of water to preserve flavor, minerals and vitamins.

It is advisable to remove visible fat and tendons before preserving or freezing. Usually, whole pieces are preserved better than the grounded ones. It is not advisable to keep the viscera because it gets easily spoiled.

For best results (except for specific cuts such as loins, roasts, legs or shoulder) it is convenient to cut or fillet the meat into individual pieces and then wrap them individually with plastic film (plastic wrap) or with foil. Subsequently, label them by type of meat and freezing date.

Make sure to freeze meat as quickly as possible in order to prevent the formation of external large ice crystals that could damage the integrity of the product. The meat can be kept frozen for up to 1 year without losing its nutrients and, especially, its texture and flavor.

How to thaw the meat

The slower the thawing takes place, the better results you will obtain. Although it might seem a waste of time, it should be started first in the refrigerator to avoid the formation of exudates (or loss of serum) that would drag off the characteristic flavors and nutrients of meat. It is also advisable not to freeze and thaw meat repeatedly because it brakes the tissues, loose nutrients and favors microbial growth. Frozen meat can also be exposed to an air stream to thaw. Then remove the exudates with a dry cloth.

After handling any type of meat

Wash your hands thoroughly with soap and warm water before and after handling poultry, fish or any other raw or frozen meat.

Cleanse well cutting boards, dishes, utensils, especially knives and work-surfaces with soap and hot water after they have been in contact with any raw meat. Place cooked food on a clean plate. If you place cooked food on an unwashed plate that have had raw meat before, bacteria from uncooked foods can contaminate cooked food.

6. Stews, root vegetables and whole grain pasta

We recommend eating 1 to 2 portions daily of one of the following options:

½ cup cooked dried vegetables or legumes
½ potato or
½ sweet potato
½ cup cooked pasta

Legumes (beans)

They are plants whose fruit is a pod. As the plant matures, the pods are dried and seeds are born. Ripe pods store food for the seed to germinate, so when ripe they contain more nutrients than when they are still mature.

While the main source of protein is meat, legumes are also rich in proteins, although with some differences:

The biological value of meat proteins is more than twice the biologic value of vegetable protein. The biological value of protein is, as we mentioned above, the relative capacity of a specific protein rich food to increase the weight of growing animals. While the protein value of the meat is 100% that of the plants is less than 45%.

Another difference is that the protein from meat is complete. To obtain an equivalent complement of essential amino acids using vegetables as a source of protein, this can only be attained by consuming a variety of vegetable products, specially the ones derived from cereal and grains, preferably whole grain, such as bread or rice.

The legumes or dried vegetables best-known and nutritive are:

dry peas
chickpeas
lima beans or butter beans (pallares)
different kinds of beans
lentils

They are rich in fiber so they help regular bowel movements. Their slowly absorbed carbohydrates provide body energy in a gradual fashion.

They are also rich in B vitamins, like thiamin and riboflavin and contain minerals such as iron and calcium.

Tubers

The **potato** is an energetic nutrient due to its high starch content. It also has a high content of water-soluble vitamins, minerals, fiber and protein.

The **sweet potato** or **boniato** is a tuber whose roots have a high content of carbohydrates, calcium, phosphorus, as well as carotene and vitamin A. Sweet potato is effective in the struggle against malnutrition due to its nutritional characteristics, ease of cultivation and productivity.

Whole grain pasta

The **pasta** is food prepared with a dough whose basic ingredient is wheat flour mixed with water. Salt, eggs or other ingredients can be added to obtain a product that is usually cooked in boiling water.

Note: The pasta and tubers are a healthy diet option, provided they are not consumed along with other high-calorie foods.

7. Red meat

Eat occasionally, 1 or 2 times a month.

The term "red meat" refers to meat derived from large beef cattle, especially cows and oxen.It also refers to bushmeat, like hare, partridge, pigeon, pheasant and quail, besides viscera, such as kidney, liver and heart.

Adult lamb or old sheep also have red meat, while those which are still suckling are considered to have white meat.

Its name is due to its color, which depends on the chemical form in which a protein, myoglobin, is present in muscle fibers. Myoglobin, is an oxygen binding protein that gets red due to its Heme-iron-oxygen constitution. This iron-heme association makes iron atoms easily absorbed. Red meat contains more purines (especially game meat and viscera) than white meat. Purines turn into uric acid and if consumed in excess can cause painful gout attacks.

Since this type of meat is the one that contains more saturated fat, it is necessary to control its intake. The fats in red meat cuts are difficult to separate from the lean meat, so the fat intake is usually higher than with other meats. The consumption of red meats and saturated fat is clearly associated to an increased cholesterol blood level.

Medical Note:
As already mentioned, excessive protein intake has no benefit to the individual. On the contrary, it can produce acidosis and bone loss, as well as it can accelerate age related renal function loss.

8. Sweets and candies

It is recommended to limit its consumption.

Sweet and candies are usually sugary delicacies intended to satisfy an immediate craving. Its consumption in excess has spread mainly in children and can trigger health problems like obesity, diabetes, caries and even anemia. Candies rarely provide Iron and cause loss of appetite when eaten instead of nutritious foods. The only nutritional values that sweets contain are refined sugars (or carbohydrates), fats of uncertain quality and little or nothing of protein, vitamins or minerals.

WEEKLY MENU & SHOPPING

Detailed information for preparing the menu

From breakfast to dinner, the menu for 30 days will show you how to have a balanced and varied combination of foods. We also include the necessary ingredients for the preparation of each recipe.

- If you need to **lose weight**, your option is a diet having a caloric value lower than what your body needs.
- If you want to **maintain weight**, your choice would be a diet specifically suited to the amount of calories your body needs.

Designing the weekly menu

It is important to broaden the group of food consumed, alternating different fruits and vegetables. We include in our weekly list of fresh vegetables and fruits, green, red, orange and yellow products. These four colors represent the presence of various beneficial substances for our body such as vitamins, minerals and antioxidants.

Taking into account these considerations allows you to draw the appropriate menu for each day of the week. You should also make a list to buy the ingredients of selected recipes.

Buying Advice

Golden rules:

- Do not buy foods you should not eat, so you will have fewer temptations at home.
- Satisfy your appetite before going to the supermarket: an empty stomach is a bad adviser during shopping.
- Start your journey by selecting vegetables and fruits from your weekly list. Filling the cart with vegetables will decrease the temptation to add other foods of little nutritional value.

Once at home, we recommend you to read the instructions in the recipes because some can be prepared in advance. For example: blanching vegetables, cooking beans, cooking chicken breasts, preparing broths and soups. Once cooked, some ingredients of the recipes can be stored refrigerated or frozen. In this way, you can save valuable time on the day you need them.

Classification of vegetables

Vegetables can be classified according to the section of the plant to which they belong. For example:

Fruits: eggplant, peppers, tomatoes and okra.
Bulbs: garlic, onion, green onion and leek.
Coles: cabbage, broccoli, cauliflower and Brussels sprouts.
Leaves: lettuce and spinach.
Peponides: zucchini, pumpkin and cucumber.
Roots: radish, beetroot and carrot.
Stem: celery, green or white asparagus, chives or chives etc.
Immature pods: green beans or green beans
Interior or stipe bole or trunk of the palm: palm

Note: edible fungi and mushrooms are usually sold in the vegetable section but they are a separate kingdom called Fungi. This is due to features such as the absence of chlorophyll and the presence of chitin, a protein that is present only in the animal kingdom.

Culinary note: many of the vegetables used in these recipes, once blanched and packed at home, can be frozen up to one year. However, our recommendation is to store them for less time to avoid losing their original taste and texture. Periods of freezing detailed in this book are due to the author's culinary criteria.

Selecting, storing and preserving fresh produce used in the recipes.

Fruits

Eggplant: choose those that are firm and heavy for their size. The tastiest are the smallest, with the skin smooth and shiny. The color, depending on the variety, must always be uniform, without spots, wrinkles or soft spots. The more mature ones tend to be large and fibrous as well as bitter.

To find out if an eggplant is ripe, make a slight finger pressure on the edge of the area near the stem, if the fingers leave an imprint, the eggplant is ripe, if after pressure marks are not present, the eggplant has not yet reached its optimum ripeness.

It is important to handle eggplant carefully and keep refrigerated for seven days. They should never be wrapped in plastic because this prevents "breathing". They should be kept isolated from the rest of vegetables and fruits, as they may deteriorate because of ethylene gas produced by respiration of the other plants.

Bell Peppers: different colors peppers are sold in the market: green, red, yellow, orange, purple, white and even black. There are about 2000 species worldwide, some of which change color from green to orange to red (sweeter taste) as they mature.

It is recommended to select the fleshy, hard and heavy specimens in proportion to their size. They should be firm and bright colored, have smooth skin, be lustrous and without bumps or bruises. The stem should be green, firm and crisp.

If the peppers have wrinkles or spots, it might mean that they have been stored for too long, causing a loss of nutrients and flavor.

Refrigerate unwashed fresh peppers in a perforated plastic bag for up to 15 days. Seared and peeled peppers can be frozen in an airtight container for up to three months.
see technique for slightly roasting peppers

Tomato: Choose tomatoes that have a firm consistency and intense defined color. The skin should be smooth with no wrinkles, cracks, or bruising. Ripe tomatoes give off a sweet aroma and are soft to touch. It is recommended to buy them semi mature because they keep on "breathing" (maturing) during storage.

If you are going to use them raw, they should be washed with abundant water. They do not need special storage conditions but can be refrigerated in the greengrocer drawer for a week. Their skin and acidity allow no significant loss of vitamins. The natural tomato juice or crushed tomatoes can be stored refrigerated for up to two days. The raw fruit is not suitable for freezing because it gets soft, but sauces and dishes prepared with tomato can be freeze up to six months.

Okra: It is recommended to choose tender or small okra, not ripe and of an intense color. It is a delicate vegetable, is better preserved in a paper bag for up to 7 days.

Previously bleached, supports up to six months frozen.

Bulbs

Garlic: the best quality, are those with small heads, firm, heavy, no sprouts and dry wrap.

The garlic should be stored in a dry, cool and well ventilated place, to prevent they get mold or begin to germinate. If you decide to separate the garlic cloves, they may be stored unpeeled, in a glass jar with holes. No freezing is allowed.

Onion: Choose those that are hard, firm and have short neck. Turn down the moist or spotted onions.

It is necessary to store in a cool dry place to keep them in good condition for several days or weeks. Once cut, they can be wrapped in plastic and refrigerated for several days. No freezing is allowed.

Green onion: It is important to note that green onions are not true bulbs but a thickening of the set of leaves at its base.

Choose the bright green stems with a delicate aroma. Its characteristic shape is long and thin. It is recommended to take only their whites and only three or four inches of the stalk; the rest should be discarded. It stays fresh in the refrigerator for 3 or 4 days.

Ciboulettes or chives: it is one of the typical "herbs" of French cuisine. The stems (leaves) should be firm, straight, smooth, dark green and shiny. They have a mild aroma and a particularly delicious taste.
It can be refrigerated in an airtight container for up to four days.

Pore: Choose white, straight and consistent stems, without marks or thick areas. The leaves must show a dark green color and a flat shape. Turn down those with yellowing leaves, soft, discolored, dry or swollen stem. Such characteristics indicate that the edible part will not have the desired consistency when cooked.

To store them, cut the stem lengthwise and wash the leaves with water. They must be separated one by one, in order to eliminate the dirt that lies between them. Pores are kept in good condition refrigerated in the greengrocer drawer for up to two weeks. Once cooked, they should be eaten within 2 days, because they can be indigestible. It is preferable not to freeze them because their texture may soften and change their flavor.

Cabbages

Cabbage: select those which are hard, crisp, compact and heavy for their size. Turn down those whose center is dry, broken, sticky or stringy and with withered leaves. Do not choose cabbages with internal leaves that are not equal to the outside leaves. This may indicate that the outer leaves have been torn out to conceal a possible lack of freshness.

When refrigerated in a perforated plastic bag, they stay fresh for 2 or 3 weeks. It is convenient to use a section isolated from other foods to avoid impregnating their intense aroma.

They can be frozen for up to three months after they have been cut and blanched. However, once thawed, they become less crisp than the fresh ones.

see technique for blanching vegetables

Broccoli: choose broccoli that has a head with small and compact clusters, uniform color, and dark green, purple or reddish green. The stem should be firm, well-cut and proportional in size. Turn down those with the flowers opened, and those that are soft or yellowish.

Broccoli can be refrigerated unwashed for up to five days in perforated plastic bags to prevent mold. If not refrigerated, it becomes fibrous and woody, developing unpleasant flavors in a short time. Once blanched, it can be frozen in an airtight container for up to three months.

see technique for blanching vegetables

Cauliflower: choose those that look clean, firm and compact, with green and tender leaves. Outbreaks should be of a creamy white color. Do not choose stained cauliflowers or with a pale color.

To store it, you should not wash until you are going to use it. Can be refrigerated wrapped in a perforated plastic bag for 1 week.

Cauliflower can also be preserved by freezing, selecting those stems that are more firm and white. Blanch previously and store in an airtight container for up to three months.

see technique for blanching vegetables

Brussels sprout: seasonal sprouts are those sold in the markets during autumn and winter.

Select those with smooth, firm, compact head and heavy for their size. The stem should be clean and white (usually sold without stem). The ones with the best taste are the small, green and hard ones, turn down those yellow or brown colored.

Do not choose sprouts showing stains or withered spots, as this indicates that they have been stored too long, thereby reducing its nutritional value and developing a slightly musty flavor.

They stay fresh unwashed in a perforated plastic bag in the greengrocer drawer of the refrigerator for 1 week.

They can be blanched and stored frozen in plastic bags or airtight containers for up to 1 year.

see technique for blanching vegetables

Leaves

Lettuce: in all its varieties, the fresher ones are distinguished by the intense color of its leaves. Once at home, immediately unpack and discard any leaves that are damaged to prevent spread of oxidation and damage to the rest.

Before use, wash the lettuce to remove pesticides traces that they may contain. To better preserve the leaves, it is recommended to remove, wash and keep them wrapped in a damp paper towel in the refrigerator for up to 8 days.

Spinach: It is recommendable to select those that look fresh, with uniform bright green color. It is advisable to turn down those with reddish or yellowish spots, because it is likely to have arisen as a result of fungal contamination. Dispose the ones with rough leaves, with a fibrous stem and those who have lost their color intensity.

Refrigerate spinach unwashed in a perforated plastic or wrapped in damp paper towel for up to two weeks.

Once blanched, it can be frozen and stored in airtight containers for up to 1 year.

see technique for blanching vegetables

Peponides

Zucchini: select zucchini firm to touch, compact, small or medium sized, having smooth spotless skin, and heavy for their size. Turn down large zucchini, because they have less tender meat and too many seeds. The intensity of green color on the skin does not affect the quality of this vegetable, since this characteristic depends on its variety.

They stay fresh by storing them unwashed in the greengrocer drawer of the refrigerator for up to two weeks. They are sensitive to contact with fruits, so it is recommended to store them isolated.

They can be frozen for up to three months after they are cut and blanched. However, once thawed they become less crisp than fresh.

see technique for blanching vegetables

Pumpkin: when selecting a pumpkin, it must be taken into account whether it is a winter or summer variety.

If you want to buy a summer pumpkin, the tenderest are those with a very soft shiny skin. If you were to buy a winter pumpkin, we recommend the heavy and mature ones, with a thick crust.

Generally, we recommend purchasing those that are firm, with intact skin. Besides, it is preferable to retain their tail or stalk to prevent pulp moisture loss.

The summer varieties are more perishable because they are full with water and their thin skin does not protect them well. These can be refrigerated in a perforated plastic bag for 1 week. After they are cut and blanched, freeze for up to 3 months. However, once thawed they are less crisp than fresh.

The winter varieties are more resistant than the summer ones due to its lower proportion of water. Their thick skin protects them. This type of pumpkin can be stored without further care for up to six months.

see technique for blanching vegetables

Cucumber: select cucumbers that show a dark green skin without yellow stains or flaws, firm, not very thick and well developed.

Avoid buying large cucumbers because they have a bitter taste, a softer texture and many hard seeds. If when pressing the stem end is felt soft, it is a sign that has been collected some time ago. Cucumber is a vegetable that should be eaten unripe, because when mature it loses its smoothness, acquires a yellowish color and its flavor becomes flattened.

Cucumbers can be kept fresh in the refrigerator for 3 or 4 days. If you need to refrigerate them after they have been cut, wrap them in plastic because they easily absorb odors. Do not tolerate extreme temperatures, so freezing is not recommended.

Roots

Radish: select medium size ones because they have a less fibrous consistency. Select those that are firm, bright red, with soft and complete skin, without fissures. If radishes preserve their leaves, they must be of an intense color to ensure their freshness. Turn down large or soft roots, and those with yellowish neck.

To retain their qualities for a long time, it is advisable to remove the green parts to avoid them getting dry. The radishes should be stored in perforated plastic bags in the refrigerator. In this way, they stay fresh for up to 7 days. It is advised not to wash them until they are to be used. Freezing is not recommended.

Beetroot: as it is a vegetable that is sold in bundles, prefer those with roots of the same size, thus all will cook uniformly.

We recommend choosing those which are smooth, firm, round, fleshy and of intense color, without spots or bruises. The selected bundles should have green leaves, as they indicate that the roots are young. However, even when the leaves are wilted or soft, beetroot is in good condition if the root is firm to touch.

It must be refrigerated leafless, unwashed, in a perforated plastic bag for up to 2 to 3 weeks. It is not advisable to freeze the raw beetroots because they soften. It is suggested to cut them into chunks, then blanch and freeze in airtight containers for up to six months.

see technique for blanching vegetables

Carrot: it can be found at the market throughout the year. Baby carrots with a good color have a delicate flavor and are ideal to eat them whole and raw. The large ones are packaged separately, and mostly used for grating or cooking.

The skin should be smooth, of a bright orange color and with a firm texture. Avoid buying flaccid carrots with wrinkles, spots, or outbreaks.

Fresh carrots do not need refrigeration when stored in a cool, fresh place. However, in case you have no adequate space, they can be refrigerated for 2-3 weeks.

Once blanched and stored in bags or airtight containers, they can be frozen for up to eight months.

see technique for blanching vegetables

Celery: choose celery with a lustrous green appearance, having a thick, compact, firm, and crisp stem, and with green colored, fresh or slightly wilted leaves. Discard the soft celeries, those with stains and dry spots, and with white superior stems or branches.

They stay in good conditions for up to 5 or 6 days wrapped in damp paper towel and properly refrigerated. Freezing is not recommended.

Asparagus: top quality asparagus, green or white, fresh or canned, can be purchased at the market. The green ones should be brightly colored and shiny; and the white ones should have a defined creamy-white color. Choose asparagus with closed and compact tips, straight and firm stem, not discolored. Discard the asparagus with bumps or bruises.

Fresh asparagus can be refrigerated wrapped in damp paper towel for up to three weeks. Keep in mind that over time they become hard, so it is best eating them as soon as possible.

If you want to freeze asparagus, you must blanch them previously. We suggest storing them in plastic bags or airtight containers, ensuring that there are no empty spaces between them. This way they will remain in good conditions for up to 1 year.

see technique for blanching vegetables

Green peas: it is a pea that includes its seeds. It is one of the most highly ranked vegetables because of their caloric value, due to its high carbohydrates and protein content. Select those with large dark green pods.

It will stay fresh in the greengrocer drawer of the refrigerator. It tolerates freezing for up to six months without being whitewashed.

Green beans: select those that present a vivid and brilliant color without discoloration, appear regular and are not too hard to touch. One way to know if they are fresh is to bend them nearing their tips to see if they break. If they do not break, they are not good. You should turn down those that are too tough and fibrous, which have passed the point of maturation. The best green beans are those in which the seeds are poorly marked.

They are kept in good condition by keeping them unwashed in a perforated plastic bag and refrigerated for 10 days.

To freeze them they must be previously blanched. To prevent seed loss, consider the following: blanch after cutting them if the cut is transverse, and blanch before cutting them if the cut is longitudinal. They can be frozen for up to three months.

see technique for blanching vegetables

Sprouts

Chinese bean: they are shoots or bean sprouts or mung beans, small stalks of tender developing roots.

Although you can refrigerate them for a few days, it is best eaten fresh to prevent rusting. Freezing is not recommended.

Buds

Palm: (heart of palm), usually sold canned, pre-cooked, or in glass containers. Most come from Brazil.

Once opened, the palm is a highly perishable food. It is recommended to remove the palm heart from the container, drain well and wrap in plastic. This can be kept refrigerated for two weeks or so.

The palm color appearance tends to fade easily in contact with air, and that is why it is not usually marketed fresh. It can not be frozen.

Mushrooms

Edible fungi and mushrooms: select them fresh, whole, small or medium sized and having good color, according to its kind. Do not pick mushrooms affected by wilting, fermentation, mold or damaged by cold.

In general, you should not dip or wash them with water, but clean them with a damp cloth or brush and dry them carefully to avoid losing their aroma.

They stay fresh for up to five days wrapped in a clean, damp cloth, refrigerated in the greengrocer drawer. The storage time depends on its initial state and consistency. Some species should be eaten freshly picked.

There are other forms of conservation which allow enjoying them for longer. However, with any of them (marinated in vinegar, oil, dried me) lose flavor and texture. To prevent the oxidation of fungi or mushrooms, cut them shortly before use. No freezing is allowed.

Fruits

How to select and store fresh fruits:

This group of edible fruits is obtained from cultivated or wild plants. Unlike plants, they have more intense flavors and aromas, as well as different nutritional properties. They should be eaten when ripe.

A ripe fruit or in point:

Smell is always the best ally to recognize if fruits are ripe or not, besides being aware of their particular characteristics.

Apricots: this fruit is so delicate that a tap with your fingernail or applying a higher pressure with your fingers damages and stains the product and leads to rapid decay.

It is recognized that the fruit is in optimal conditions if you notice a soft consistency when pressed gently between two fingers.

Preferably, eat the apricots just right. You can keep it refrigerated for 3 or 4 days in a perforated plastic bag. Thereafter, the skin becomes wrinkled and the pulp gets dry.

Cherry: It is recommended to choose those dark red colored, heavy for their size, with a shiny skin, having firm consistency, and fresh green stems.
Ideally, consume them immediately, but can be refrigerated unwashed for up to 7 days.

Plum:

The yellow plums are fruits with a citrus flavor, and with abundant juice.

The red plums are juicy and sweeter than the yellow ones.

The black plums have a bluish or blackish skin, and are best suited for baking or making compote.
When you choose plums, make sure they are firm, not bruised, and covered with a light opaque dust.

If you buy green plums, leave them at room temperature until ripe. Refrigerated, they only stay fresh for 3 or 4 days, as they lose moisture and the skin becomes wrinkled with time.

Berries: Buy ripe fruits because they do not ripen at home. Choose those with an intense and brilliant color, not too soft, without bumps or bruises.

In gastronomy, considered berries are the following:

Blueberry
Cranberry
Raspberry
Strawberry
Blackberry
Elderberry
Dewberry

To keep the berries at room temperature, place them in an airtight container without washing them, in a single layer. The raspberries, blackberries and blueberries, become deteriorate in 2 or 3 days. Elderberries are kept fresh for 4 or 5 days, while blueberries are kept fresh up to 1 week.

If you prefer to refrigerate them, place a single layer of unwashed fruit in an open container, covered with a damp cloth.

Strawberry: it is mentioned separately because it is one of the most popular berries. Select those that look fresh, firm and thick, without blows, bright and well-red colored. They are delicate and perishable, and must be purchased with intact stems. Do not remove the stems until they are ready for washing, in order to keep them tasty.

We recommend washing them by placing the berries in a colander under running soft water. To dry them, place them on paper towel and remove the stem with pliers.

Strawberries are better preserved when stored in the refrigerator or in a cool, dark, ventilated place, scattered as possible, in a serving dish. If they are not quite ripe, they can be maintained in good conditions for up to 4 or 5 days. XXX

Fig: Unlike other fruits, wrinkles and openings in the fig's skin show they are at the ideal time to consume them because it is evidence that the fruit has reached its maturity.
They should have a nice color, good consistency and relatively smooth texture. When ripe, they yield to gentle pressure with your fingers. It is convenient to discard the fruits if they are hard and shriveled, with bitter odor or flattened sides. XXX

The figs are very delicate, making it difficult to market them. Even when they are stored in the refrigerator, they require special care and are kept only for 3 days.

Lemon: among the most common are the following:

The acid lime or Galician lime (*Citrus aurantifolia*), also known as Mexican lemon, **Peruvian lemon**, Creole lemon or Pica lemon. The fruit is round or oval, small, with yellowish-green skin, with seeds, and sometimes with a small nipple.

The **Eureka lemon** (*Citrus limon*) has spherical or oblong shape and has an apex shaped lump on both ends. The rind is yellow and contains glands that carry essential oils, which give them their characteristic odor.

The **sweet lemon** (*Citrus limetta*), also called lemon of Rome, sweet lime, lime Chichona or lime bergamot. It is distinguished mainly by its very low astringency and its characteristic nipples at both ends.

The **Persian or Tahiti lime** (*Citrus latifolia*), Persian lime, creole lemon, messina lemon or seeded lemon, is less acidic than the others, larger and seeded.

Generally, should be chosen the ones that are heavier for their size, smooth-skinned, firm, bright and of an intense color. Turn down soft or dried ones.

They can be kept at room temperature for one week. They can also be maintained in good conditions in the refrigerator for up to 1 month. (Be careful with very cold temperature, because they can dry).

Tangerine: like all citrus, if they are juicy they should be heavy, so it is appropriate to select those that have a greater weight with respect to their size. The best are those with soft skin, but not wrinkled and firmly attached to the segments. The stem should be cut flush. The best indicator of quality is its smell, which is sweeter and more intense when the fruit is ripe.

Tangerines can be kept in good conditions for several weeks in the warmest part of the refrigerator.

Mango: this fruit is in optimal conditions when is flexible to touch but without yielding under your finger pressure. Mangoes must be purchased when they emit a good aroma. If you buy them too green, the fruit does not ripen properly. If they have black areas, they may be past. Sometimes, mango has an outward appearance with spots and wrinkles but the flesh is in perfect conditions. The opposite happens in mango with an excellent external appearance, but with a defective pulp.

Preferably, eat the fruit while ripe. The ripe mango can be refrigerated up to 5 days.

Apple: there are several varieties. The flesh should always be firm and aromatic. Turn down those with bumps, rot, wrinkles, soft parts, or uneven spots. Some perfectly healthy varieties have dark spots or a mottled appearance. These imperfections can be found throughout the skin and are one of the characteristics of excellent specimens for use in the kitchen.

The apples stay fresh at room temperature for 1 or 2 weeks. There are varieties that stay fresh for six months or more. They tolerate refrigeration for several weeks without loss of internal moisture.

Melon or Cantaloupe: choose melons that are hard and have no markings. The ones with very green skin were collected early. When ripe, they have a very characteristic sweet and delicate smell. If they have no fragrance, let them ripen at home, at room temperature, for a few days.

To know if a melon is ripe, take it in your hands firmly. If it yields while pressing gently the extremes, it is a sign that it is ripe. Melons that are too mature may be sticky to touch. If possible, shake slightly before buying the melon: if you hear the crack of seeds, is a sign that is too old and has started to deteriorate.

The ripe fruit should be consumed immediately. The melon chilled a few hours before serving is very refreshing.

Peach: select the entire fruit, without bruises, with a uniform yellow color. Its smell should be smooth and aromatic. If chosen while still green, let them ripen for a few days at room temperature.

When mature it is advisable to keep them refrigerated separately from other fruits.

Orange: choose the heaviest in terms of size to ensure they are juicy and are at their ripest moment. Turn down the fruit with blows, bruises, or those that have a rancid smell. The skin color does not indicate quality, as there are ripe oranges with green skin. Oranges that are sold in nets are often class I and II, while the extra class is stored in wooden boxes and some are even wrapped in tissue paper.

If the oranges are to be eaten shortly, they can stay in a fruit bowl at room temperature. However, to keep them fresh, they should be refrigerated up to 1 or 2 weeks.

Avocado: make sure the skin has no stains, black spots or excessive signs of maturation. The avocado is ripe if when shaking the bone is moved or the flesh yields to gentle finger pressure.

If it is not ripe, leave at room temperature for a while. The process of maturation can be accelerated if wrapped in newspaper. If the fruit is purchased mature, the maturing process can be stopped refrigerating them for up to three days.

Note: This fruit, unlike others that are usually served as desserts, are used mainly in salads, sauces and other more elaborate recipes.

Pear: choose the fruits of uniform color, with smooth and firm skin. If they are ready or mature, they yield to gentle finger pressure.

The pear is a delicate fruit; it is advisable to remove its packaging, and store them in a cool, dry place, protected from light. You can refrigerate it for up to three days.

Pineapple: the flavor should be sweet, and the skin, uniform and clean. The skin should not yield under finger pressure, which indicates that it is too mature. Do not select the fruit if the end of the stem is moldy or stained.

The pineapple is a very fragile fruit, sensitive to temperature changes. It can be kept for several days in a cool, dry place. When peeled, the pineapple must be kept protected with plastic in the refrigerator and eaten as soon as possible.

Banana: select the fruit intact, without blows or bruises. The yellow color of the skin is indicative of the fruit maturity. Turn down those that are too soft.

Bananas do not require special storage conditions. They should be kept in a cool and dry place, protected from direct sunlight. The best way to keep them fresh is hanging them in bunches.

When they are refrigerated, peel darkens without affecting them. You can freeze them shelled in airtight containers for up to two months.

Watermelon: when the melon is ripe, it emits a hollow sound when tapped with your fingers or the palms of your hands. If you buy watermelon pieces, ensure that the meat is firm and juicy.

They can be stored fresh at room temperature for 5 days. However, refrigerated is very refreshing.

Grapefruit: choose fruits heavier for their size. Discard those with parts too hard or too soft on the skin. Grapefruit in good conditions must firmly resist finger pressure.

The grapefruits are kept in good conditions at room temperature or in refrigerator for up to 1 or 2 weeks.

Grapes: The clusters should be solid and the fruit firm, with smooth skin, and uniform size and color.

They should be washed before refrigerated. They will be kept in good conditions for up to 10 days. To maintain its flavor and aroma, it is preferable to take them off the refrigerator 1 hour before use.

Certified organic food

Organic fruits and vegetables are those in which no fertilizers or pesticides were used during production. They lack chemical preservatives and therefore their storage time is shorter. They are sold in specialized places and at a higher price than their counterpart.

30 DAY MENU SUGGESTION

OPTIONS FOR BREAKFAST
1. 1/2 cup fruit juice or 1/2 cup chopped fruit *
2. 1/2 cup whole grain cereal or 1/4 cup of skim milk or nonfat yogurt *
3. 2 whole-wheat toasts with 1/2 teaspoon diet jam or 2 whole-wheat toasts with hard-boiled or boiled egg *
* 1 cup of coffee, tea or infusions with 2 teaspoons of splenda or brown sugar

DAY 1	
Lunch	**Vegetable omelet** * or **Ham or turkey sandwich** (lettuce and tomato included) *
Dinner	**Chicken sauté with vegetables** and **Brown rice with vegetables** or **Chicken sauté with vegetables** and **Country-style mashed potatoes**
	* ♀ can double the recipe with 1 single yolk
	* ♀ up to 2 units

DAY 2	
Lunch	**Broccoli crêpe** * or **Tuna sandwich**
Dinner	**Cream of vegetable soup**
	Baked chicken with Rosemary and **Baby spinach salad** or
	Baked chicken with Rosemary and **Spinach and mushroom salad in soy sauce**
	* ♀ can double the recipe with 1 single yolk

DAY 3	
Lunch	**Cherry tomato and nut salad** * or **Caprese sandwich** *
Dinner	**Chicken breast broth**
	Chicken burgers with **Hot vegetables** (1 or 2 units) * or
	Chicken burgers with **Asparagus and broccoli salad**
	* ♀ can double the recipe
	* ♀ can double the recipe
	* ♀ 2 or 3 units

DAY 4	
Lunch	**Spinach and mushrooms soufflé** * or **Tomato and avocado sandwich**
Dinner	**Baked fish in papillote** with **Brown rice** or **Baked fish in papillote** with **Baked potato with olive oil** or **Potatoes with parsley**
	* ♀ can double the recipe with 1 single yolk

DAY 5	
Lunch	**Natural-style tuna** with 4 whole grain or water crackers * or **Tuna Sandwich** *
Dinner	**Cream of mushroom soup**
	Spaghetti with vegetables and olives
	* ♀ can double the recipe
	* ♀ up to 2 units

DAY 6	
Lunch	**Chicken, asparagus and apple salad** * or **Chicken sandwich** *
Dinner	**Eggplant a la Bolognese** with **Brown rice**
	* ♀ can double the recipe
	* ♀ up to 2 units

DAY 7	
Lunch	**Spinach and mushrooms soufflé** * or **Ham sandwich** *
Dinner	**Curry chicken with mint** with **Avocado, lettuce and tomato salad**
	* ♀ can double the recipe with 1 single yolk
	* ♀ up to 2 units

DAY 8	
Lunch	**Chick-peas and sprout salad** or **Turkey sandwich** *
Dinner	**Chicken breast broth**
	Chicken Milanese (1 or 2 units) * with **Hot vegetables**
	* ♀ up to 2 units
	* ♀ 2 or 3 units

DAY 9	
Lunch	**Eggplant, peppers and rosemary salad** * or **Ham sandwich** *
Dinner	**Mediterranean salmon** with **Brown rice** and **Spinach purée**
	* ♀ can double the recipe
	* ♀ up to 2 units

DAY 10	
Lunch	**Vegetable omelet** * or **Turkey sandwich** *
Dinner	**Pork loin with sage** with **Glazed carrots** or **Pork loin with sage** with **Cabbage, carrot and raisin Chinese salad**
	* ♀ can double the recipe with 1 single yolk
	* ♀ up to 2 units

DAY 11	
Lunch	**Avocado, lettuce and tomato salad** * or **Caprese sandwich** *
Dinner	**Turkey burger** (1 or 2 units) * with **Spinach and mushrooms soufflé**
	* ♀ can double the recipe
	* ♀ up to 2 units
	* ♀ up to 2 or 3 units

DAY 12	
Lunch	**Cauliflower Crêpe** * or **Tuna sandwich** *
Dinner	**Chicken Milanese** with **Neapolitan-style mushrooms** (1 or 2 units) *
	* ♀ can double the recipe with 1 single yolk
	* ♀ up to 2 units
	* ♀ up to 2 or 3 units

DAY 13	
Lunch	**Cheese omelet** * or **Tomato and avocado sandwich** *
Dinner	**Cream of mixed vegetable soup**
	Neapolitan-style baked chicken with **Brown rice**
	* ♀ can double the recipe with 1 single yolk
	* ♀ up to 2 units

DAY 14	
Lunch	**Olive, pepper and cottage cheese salad** * or **Olive and hard-boiled egg sandwich** *
Dinner	**Chicken breast broth**
	Lentils with vegetables with 1/2 breast **Curry chicken with mint**
	* ♀ can double the recipe
	* ♀ up to 2 units with 1 single yolk

DAY 15	
Lunch	**Pepper crêpe** * or **Egg and chive sandwich** *
Dinner	**Cream of mixed vegetable soup**
	Baked fish in papillote with **Spinach and mushrooms soufflé** and **Brown rice**
	* ♀ can double the recipe with 1 single yolk
	* ♀ up to 2 units with 1 single yolk

DAY 16	
Lunch	**Vegetable omelet** * or **Chicken sandwich** *
Dinner	**Cream of mushroom soup**
	Macaroni with tofu and mushrooms
	* ♀ can double the recipe with 1 single yolk
	* ♀ up to 2 units

DAY 17	
Lunch	**Heart of palm and sun-dried tomato salad** * or **Tomato and avocado sandwich** and 1 hard-boiled egg *
Dinner	**Grilled fish** with **Spinach and mushroom salad in soy sauce** and **Brown rice**
	* ♀ can double the recipe
	* ♀ up to 2 units with 1 single yolk

DAY 18	
Lunch	**Chick-peas and sprout salad** or **Turkey sandwich** *
Dinner	**Chicken breast broth**
	Baked chicken with Rosemary, Zucchini with mushrooms au gratin and **Spinach purée**
	* ♀ up to 2 units

DAY 19	
Lunch	**Green bean Crêpe** * or **Tuna sandwich** *
Dinner	**Tomato and thyme soup**
	Baked fish in papillote with **Brown rice** and **Potatoes with parsley**
	* ♀ can double the recipe
	* ♀ up to 2 units

DAY 20	
Lunch	**Ham omelet** * or **Caprese sandwich** *
Dinner	**Cream of mixed vegetable soup**
	Spaghetti with vegetables and olives
	* ♀ can double the recipe with 1 single yolk
	* ♀ up to 2 units

DAY 21	
Lunch	**Natural-style tuna** with **avocado, lettuce and tomato salad** * or **Chicken sandwich** *
Dinner	**Tomato and thyme soup**
	Mediterranean salmon with **brown rice**
	* ♀ can double the recipe with 1 single yolk
	* ♀ up to 2 units

DAY 22	
Lunch	**Cheese crêpe** * or **Salmon sandwich** *
Dinner	**Baked fish in papillote** with **Spinach and mushrooms soufflé** and **Potatoes with parsley**
	* ♀ can double the recipe with 1 single yolk
	* ♀ up to 2 units

DAY 23	
Lunch	**Cheese omelet** * or **Ham sandwich** *
Dinner	**Lentils** with **Avocado, lettuce and tomato salad**
	* ♀ can double the recipe with 1 single yolk
	* ♀ up to 2 units

DAY 24	
Lunch	**Chick-peas and sprout salad** * or **Tuna sandwich** *
Dinner	**Cream of mushroom soup**
	Chicken sauté with vegetables and **Country-style mashed potatoes**
	* ♀ can double the recipe with 1 single yolk
	* ♀ up to 2 units

DAY 25	
Lunch	Cherry tomato and nut salad * or Tomato and avocado sandwich *
Dinner	Mediterranean salmon with Brown rice
	* ♀ can double the recipe
	* ♀ up to 2 units with 1 single yolk

DAY 26	
Lunch	Ham omelet * or Caprese sandwich *
Dinner	Macaroni with tofu and mushrooms
	* ♀ up to 2 units with 1 single yolk
	* ♀ up to 2 units

DAY 27	
Lunch	Vegetable omelet * or Olive and hard-boiled egg sandwich *
Dinner	Neapolitan-style baked chicken with Brown rice or Neapolitan-style baked chicken with Potatoes with parsley
	* ♀ up to 2 units with 1 single yolk
	* ♀ up to 2 units with 1 egg

DAY 28	
Lunch	Green bean crêpe * or Tomato and avocado sandwich *
Dinner	Baked fish in papillote with Brown rice
	* ♀ can double the recipe with 1 single yolk
	* ♀ up to 2 units with 1 egg

DAY 29	
Lunch	Pepper and mushrooms omelet * or Caprese sandwich
Dinner	Neapolitan-style baked chicken with Backed potato
	* ♀ can double the recipe with 1 single yolk
	* ♀ up to 2 units

DAY 30	
Lunch	Natural-style tuna with crackers * or Salmon sandwich *
Dinner	Turkey Milanese with Spinach purée or Brown rice
	* ♀ can double the recipe with 1 single yolk
	* ♀ up to 2 units

RECIPES

Although the recipes in this book are simple and easy to prepare, we believe that personal curiosity and creativity also play a very important role in their preparation and flavor.

The dishes shown in these pictures have been artistically presented so that the experience of adopting new eating habits turns out to be more pleasant.

The main purpose of our book is to provide as many tips as possible to help people who want and need to make healthy changes in their lifestyle.

Degree of difficulty in recipes:

1 very easy to prepare
2 easy to prepare
3 more elaborated

FIRST COURSES AND APPETIZERS

1. ***NATURAL-STYLE TUNA***
2. ***NAPOLITAN-STYLE MUSHROOMS***
3. ***BROCCOLI CRÊPE***
   Cauliflower Crêpe
   Pepper Crêpe
   Green bean Crêpe
4. ***VEGETABLE OMELET***
   Mushroom Omelet
   Turkey ham Omelet
   Cheese Omelet
5. ***VEGETABLES IN COLD OREGANO DIP***
6. ***POKER OF VEGETABLES À LA CRÉME***
7. ***SPINACH AND MUSHROOM SOUFFLÉ***

SIDES

1. ***BROWN RICE WITH VEGETABLES***
2. ***HOT VEGETABLES***
3. ***BAKED OR GRILLED POTATO***
4. ***POTATOES WITH PARSLEY***
5. ***SMALL BAKED POTATOES WITH OLIVE OIL***
6. ***SPINACH PURÉE***
7. ***COUNTRY-STYLE MASHED POTATOES***
8. ***GLAZED CARROTS***

SALADS

1. CABBAGE, CARROT AND RAISIN CHINESE SALAD
2. OLIVE, PEPPER AND COTTAGE CHEESE SALAD
3. EGGPLANT, PEPPER AND ROSEMARY SALAD
4. ASPARAGUS AND BROCCOLI SALAD
5. BABY SPINACH SALAD
6. SPINACH AND MUSHROOM SALAD IN SOY SAUCE
7. CHICK-PEAS AND SPROUT SALAD
8. HEART OF PALM AND SUNDRIED TOMATO SALAD
9. AVOCADO, LETTUCE AND TOMATO SALAD
10. CHICKEN, ASPARAGUS AND APPLE SALAD
11. CHERRY TOMATO AND NUT SALAD
12. MIXED GREEN VEGETABLE, FETA CHEESE AND PECAN

SOUPS AND CRÈMES

1. CAPRESE SANDWICH
2. OLIVE AND HARD-BOILED EGG SANDWICH
3. TUNA SANDWICH
4. EGG AND CHIVE SANDWICH
5. TURKEY OR HAM SANDWICH
6. CHICKEN SANDWICH
7. SALMON SANDWICH
8. TOMATO AND AVOCADO SANDWICH
9. HAM AND CHEESE SANDWICH

SANDWICHES

1. CAPRESE SANDWICH
2. OLIVE AND HARD-BOILED EGG SANDWICH
3. TUNA SANDWICH
4. EGG AND CHIVE SANDWICH
5. TURKEY OR HAM SANDWICH
6. CHICKEN SANDWICH
7. SALMON SANDWICH
8. TOMATO AND AVOCADO SANDWICH
9. HAM AND CHEESE SANDWICH

MAIN COURSES

1. EGGPLANT ALLA BOLOGNESE (ITALIAN)
2. CHICKEN OR TURKEY BURGER
3. CHICKEN OR TURKEY CUTLETS
4. CURRIED CHICKEN WITH MINT
5. BAKED CHICKEN WITH ROSEMARY
6. NAPOLITAN-STYLE BAKED CHICKEN
7. CHICKEN SAUTÉ WITH VEGETABLES
8. GRILLED OR BAKED FISH IN PAPILLOTE
9. GRILLED FISH
10. MEDITERRANEAN SALMON
11. EGGPLANT WITH OLIVES AU GRATE
12. PORK LOIN WITH SAGE
13. LENTILS WITH VEGETABLES
17. MACARONI WITH TOFU AND MUSHROOMS
18. SPAGHETTI WITH VEGETABLES AND OLIVES
19. ZUCCHINI WITH MUSHROOMS AU GRATIN

SALAD DRESSINGS AND SAUCES

1. PEPPER OIL
2. LEMON DRESSING
3. HOMEMADE MAYONNAISE
4. HOMEMADE MAYONNAISE WITH CURRY
5. BASIC TOMATO SAUCE
6. SWEET AND SOUR VINAIGRETTE
7. MUSTARD VINAIGRETTE

DESSERTS AND DRINKS

1. SWEET POTATO A L'ORANGE
2. FRUITS WITH YOGURT, HONEY AND ASSORTED SEEDS
3. ORANGE, CINNAMON AND CLOVE GELATIN
4. STRAWBERRY FRAPPÉ
5. FROZEN LEMONADE
6. HOT OR ICED GREEN TEA WITH LEMON
7. HOT OR ICED GREEN TEA WITH MINT AND GINGER

FIRST COURSES AND APPETIZERS

1. NATURAL-STYLE TUNA

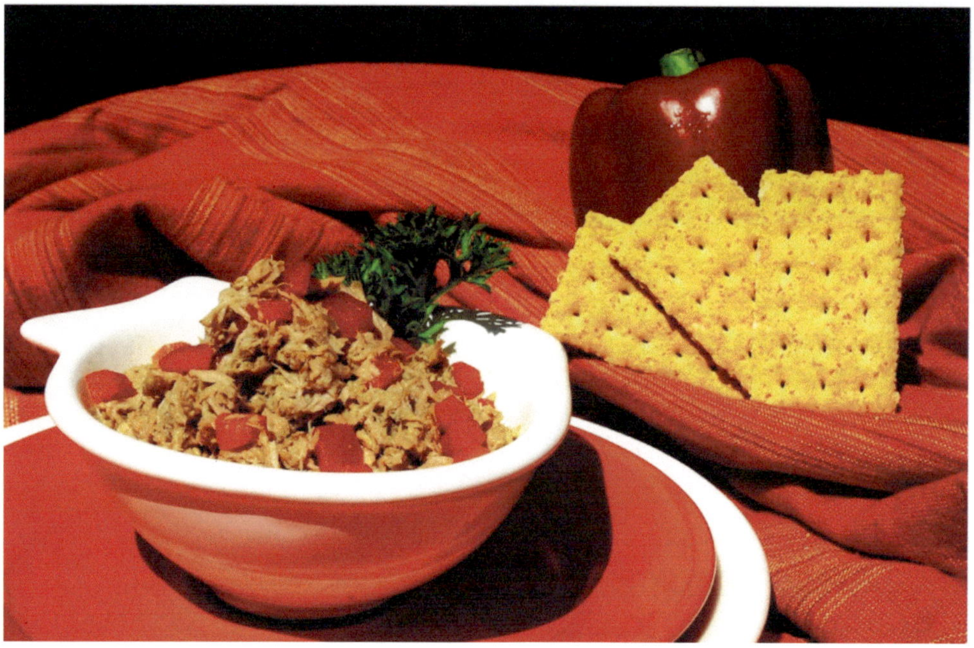

Serves 1
Preparation time: 10 minutes
Degree of difficulty: 1

1	NATURAL-STYLE TUNA			
	Ingredients for 1 portion	**Equivalences**		**Calories**
▪	1 tuna can, packed in water	130 g	4.5 oz	144.00
▪	¼ cup raw red bell pepper peeled and diced			20.80
▪	½ tablespoon Dijon mustard			0.00
▪	1 tablespoon balsamic vinegar			12.00
▪	1 tablespoon extra virgin olive oil*			134.00
▪	a pinch of salt and pepper			0.40
	* or any other gourmet oil of your choice	**Total Calories**		**311.20**

→ Open the can tuna and drain liquid. → Empty contents into a salad bowl. → Mix well with mustard, vinegar and oil. → Form a uniform mixture. → Add diced peppers and mix. → Serve cold with a salad or potatoes with parsley. → Can be used as an appetizer with whole wheat crackers or toast. → Keep refrigerated.

2. NEAPOLITAN-STYLE MUSHROOMS

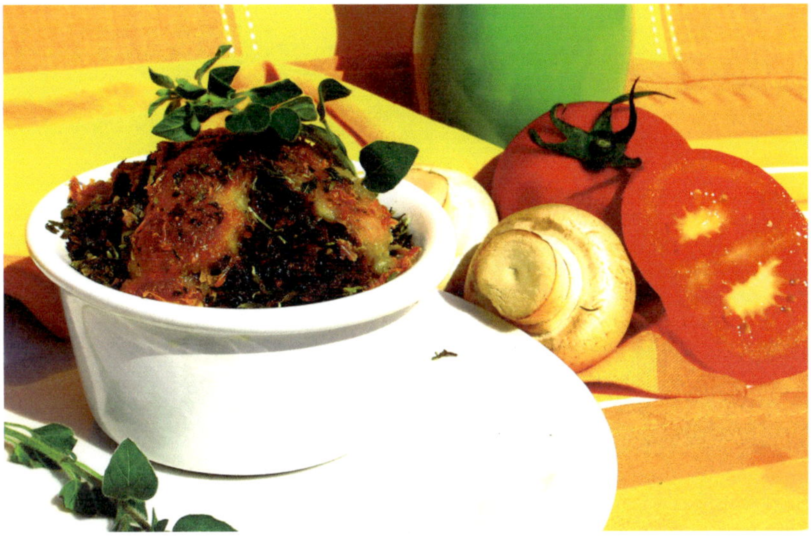

Serves 2
Preparation time: 15 minutes
Degree of difficulty: 2

2	NAPOLITAN-STYLE MUSHROOMS			
	Ingredients for 2 portions	Equivalences		Calories
■	2 cups fresh mushrooms, diced			33.28
■	1 medium-sized onion, diced	½	cup	8.15
■	4 tomatoes peeled, seeded and diced			18.12
■	½ cup fresh low fat mozzarella cheese, shredded			90.00
■	1 teaspoon minced garlic			5.70
■	1 tablespoon dried oregano			0.00
■	1 tablespoon extra virgin olive or avocado oil			134.00
■	a pinch of salt and pepper			0.40
		Total Calories		**289.65**

Preheat oven to 390º F - 200º C.

→ Heat oil in a non-stick frying pan. → Add onion and fry for 1 minute. → Add garlic and brown slightly. → Add mushrooms and stir for a few minutes, then add diced tomatoes. → Season with salt and pepper.

→ Remove from heat and place in a small baking dish. → Add shredded mozzarella cheese. → Sprinkle with oregano. → Bake for 5 minutes or until cheese is *bubbly*. → Garnish with a sprig of fresh oregano. → Serve warm..

see frying
see browning
see gratinéing

3. BROCCOLI CRÊPE

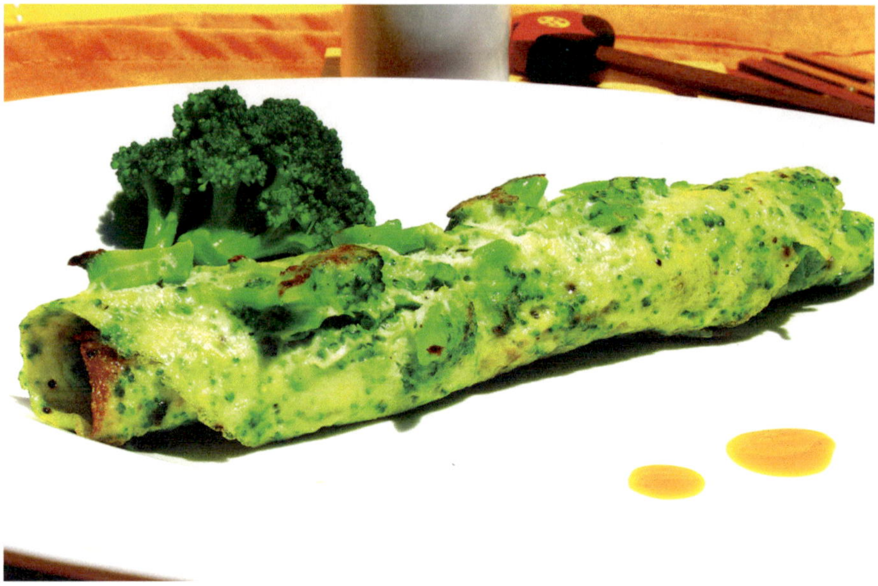

Serves 2
Preparation time: 8 minutes
Degree of difficulty: 2

3	BROCCOLI CRÊPE			
	Ingredients for 2 portions	Equivalences		Calories
▪	1 cup broccoli florets, cut into small pieces			17.97
▪	2 eggs, preferably *Omega-3* egg			180.00
▪	½ tablespoon extra virgin olive or avocado oil			67.00
▪	a pinch of salt and pepper			0.40
		Total Calories		**265.37**

→ Blanch broccoli. → Drain excess water. → Set aside. → Beat eggs slightly in a bowl using a fork. → Add broccoli. → Season with salt and pepper and mix well. → Set aside. → Heat oil in a non-stick frying pan. → Add preparation and fry. → Form a crêpe and brown slightly on both sides. → Roll and serve warm.

see blanching vegetables
see frying
see browning

Variations of Broccoli Crêpe

- Cauliflower Crêpe:

Serves 2
Preparation time: 8 minutes
Degree of difficulty: 2

-	**Cauliflower Crêpe**			
	Ingredients for 2 portions	**Equivalences**		**Calories**
▪	½ cup cauliflower florets, cut into small pieces			11.10
▪	2 eggs, preferably *Omega-3* egg			180.00
▪	½ tablespoon extra virgin olive or avocado oil			67.00
▪	a pinch of salt and pepper			0.40
		Total Calories		**258.50**

→ Blanch cauliflower. → Drain excess water. → Set aside. → Beat eggs slightly in a bowl using a fork. → Add cauliflower. → Season with salt and pepper and mix well. → Set aside. → Heat oil in a non-stick frying pan. → Add preparation and fry. → Form a crêpe and brown slightly on both sides. → Roll and serve warm.
.

see blanching vegetables
see frying
see browning

- *Pepper Crêpe:*

Serves 2
Preparation time: 8 minutes
Degree of difficulty: 2

-	**Pepper Crêpe**			
	Ingredients for 2 portions	**Equivalences**		**Calories**
■	½ cup red bell pepper, cut into small pieces			10.40
■	2 eggs, preferably *Omega-3* egg			180.00
■	½ tablespoon extra-virgin olive or avocado oil			67.00
■	a pinch of salt and pepper			0.40
		Total Calories		**257.80**

→ Blanch pepper. → Drain excess water. → Set aside. → Beat eggs slightly in a bowl using a fork. → Add pepper. → Season with salt and pepper and mix well. → Set aside. → Heat oil in a non-stick frying pan. → Add preparation and fry. → Form a crêpe and brown slightly on both sides. → Roll and serve warm.

see blanching vegetables
see frying
see browning

- Green Bean Crêpe:

Serves 2
Preparation time: 8 minutes
Degree of difficulty: 2

-	Green bean Crêpe			
	Ingredients for 2 portions	Equivalences		Calories
▪	½ cup green bean, cut into small pieces			14.30
▪	2 eggs, preferably *Omega-3* egg			180.00
▪	½ tablespoon extra-virgin olive or avocado oil			67.00
▪	a pinch of salt and pepper			0.40
		Total Calories		**261.70**

→ Blanch green bean. → Drain excess water. → Set aside. → Beat eggs slightly in a bowl using a fork. → Add green bean. → Season with salt and pepper and mix well. → Set aside. → Heat oil in a non-stick frying pan. → Add preparation and fry. → Form a crêpe and brown slightly on both sides. → Roll and serve warm.

see blanching vegetables
see frying
see browning

4. VEGETABLE OMELET

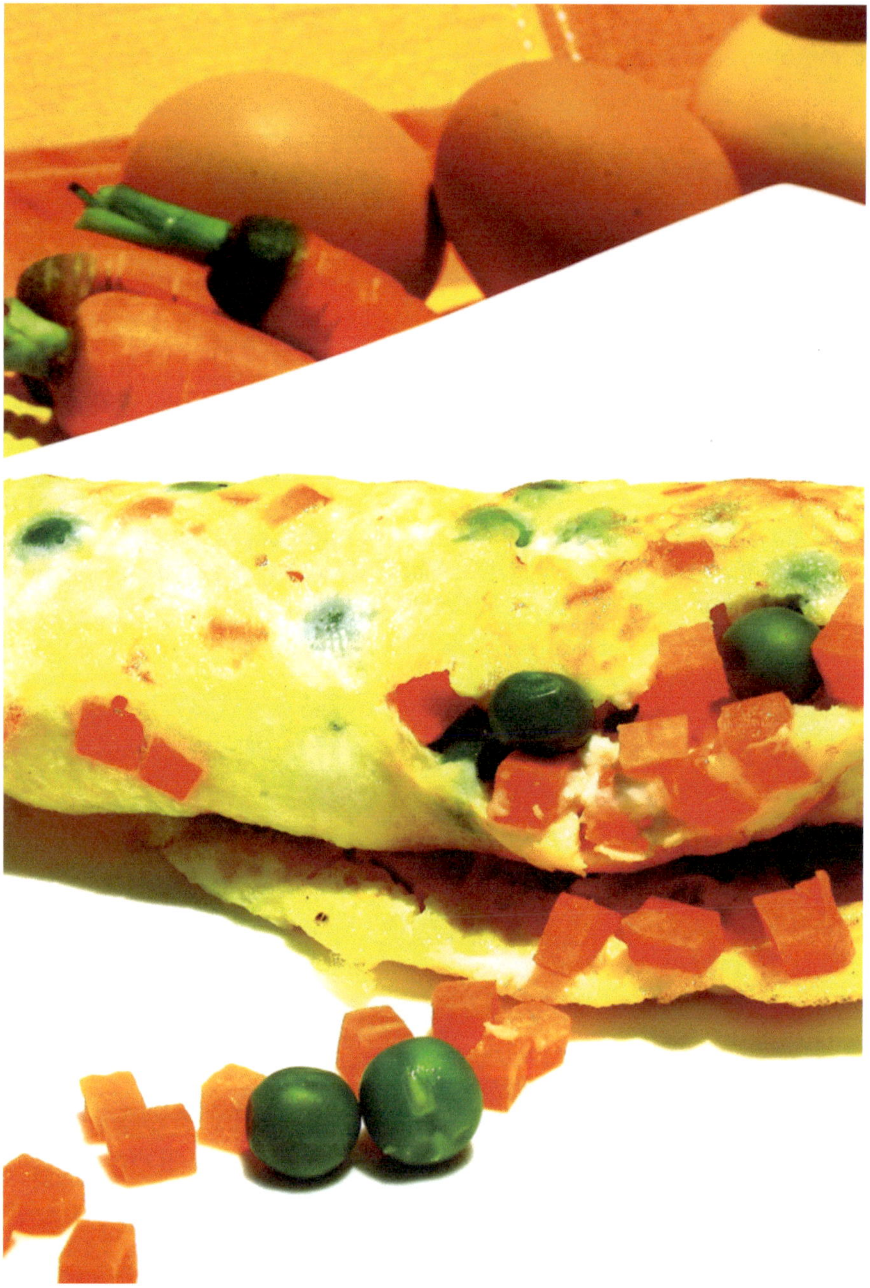

Serves 2
Preparation time: 10 minutes
Degree of difficulty: 2

4	VEGETABLE OMELET			
	Ingredients for 2 portions	**Equivalences**		**Calories**
▪	¼ cup peas, blanched			18.50
▪	¼ cup carrots, minced and blanched			19.00
▪	2 eggs, preferably *Omega-3* egg			180.00
▪	1 tablespoon, low-fat feta cheese			30.00
▪	1 tablespoon extra virgin olive or avocado oil			134.00
▪	a pinch of salt and pepper			0.40
		Total Calories		**381.90**

→ Beat eggs in a bowl. → Add cheese and blanched and drained vegetables. → Season with salt and pepper. → Heat oil in a non-stick frying pan. → Fry ingredients creating a thin omelet. → Fold the egg mixture in half forming the omelet. → Serve warm.

see blanching vegetables
see frying

Variations to vegetable omelet:

- *Mushroom Omelet*

Serves 2
Preparation time: 10 minutes
Degree of difficulty: 2

-	Mushroom Omelet			
	Ingredients for 2 portions	**Equivalences**		**Calories**
▪	1 cup raw mushroom, sliced			16.64
▪	2 eggs, preferably *Omega-3* egg			180.00
▪	1 tablespoon extra virgin olive or avocado oil			134.00
▪	a pinch of salt and pepper			0.40
		Total Calories		**331.04**

→ Beat eggs in a bowl. → Add mushrooms. → Season with salt and pepper. → Heat oil in a non-stick frying pan. → Fry ingredients creating a thin omelet. → Fold the egg mixture in half forming the omelet. → Serve warm.

see frying

- *Turkey or Ham Omelet*

Serves 2
Preparation time: 10 minutes
Degree of difficulty: 2

-	Turkey Ham Omelet			
	Ingredients for 2 portions	**Equivalences**		**Calories**
▪	2 shaved lean deli meat (turkey or ham), minced	40 g	1.4 oz	38.40
▪	2 eggs, preferably *Omega-3* egg			180.00
▪	1 tablespoon extra virgin olive or avocado oil			134.00
▪	a pinch of salt and pepper			0.40
		Total Calories		**382.80**

→ Beat eggs in a bowl. → Add turkey or ham. → Season with salt and pepper. → Heat oil in a non-stick frying pan. →Fry ingredients, creating a thin omelet. → Fold in half forming the omelet. → Serve warm.

see frying

- *Cheese Omelet*

Serves 2
Preparation time: 10 minutes
Degree of difficulty: 2

-	**Cheese Omelet**			
	Ingredients for 2 portions	**Equivalences**		**Calories**
▪	2 eggs, preferably *Omega-3* egg			180.00
▪	1 tablespoon crumbled low fat ricotta cheese			12.50
▪	1 tablespoon extra virgin olive or avocado oil			134.00
▪	a pinch of salt and pepper			0.40
		Total Calories		**326.90**

→ Beat eggs in a bowl. → Add ricotta cheese. → Season with salt and pepper. → Heat oil in a non-stick frying pan. → Fry ingredients creating a thin omelet. → Fold in half forming the omelet. → Serve warm.

see frying

5. VEGETABLES IN COLD OREGANO SAUCE

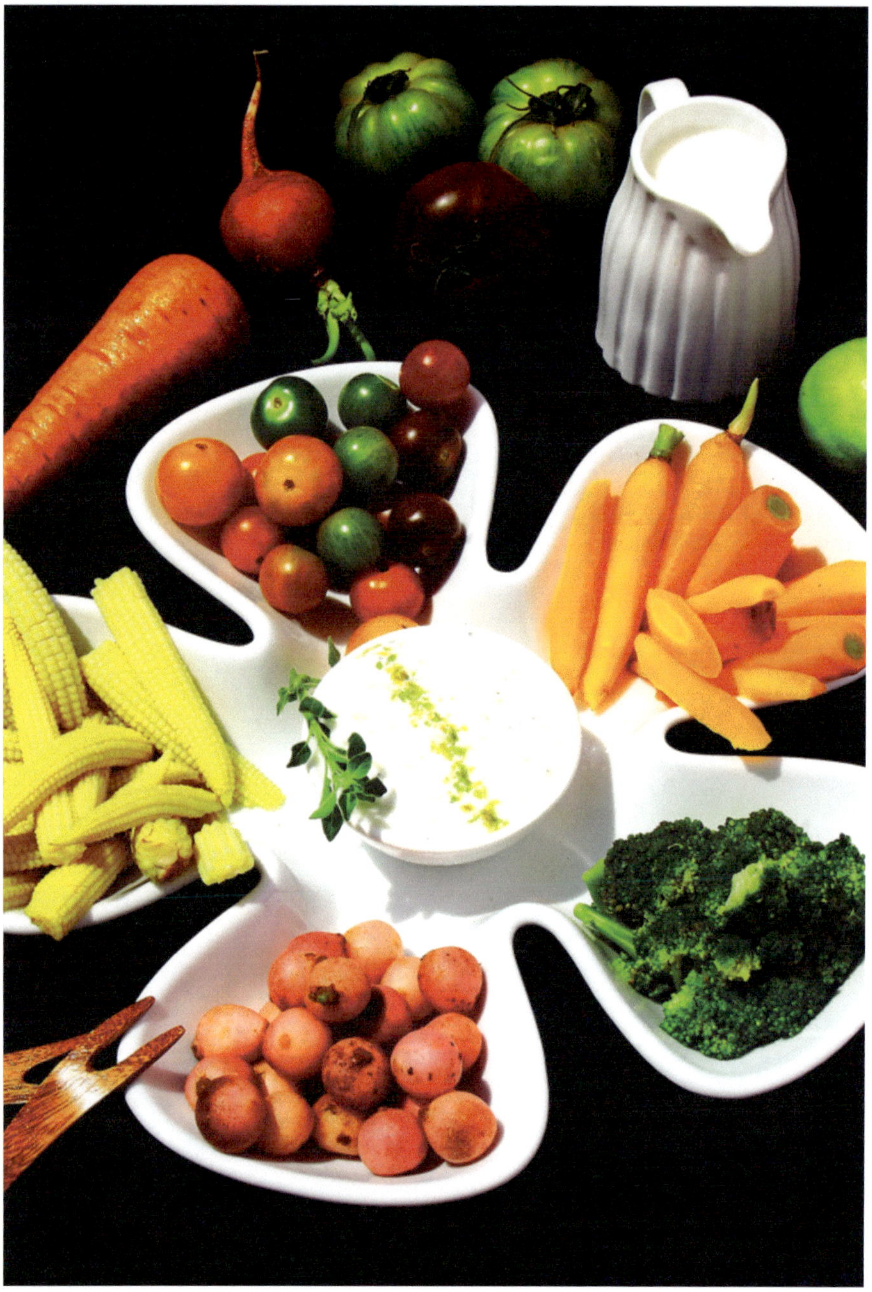

Serves 2-4
Preparation time: 30 minutes
Degree of difficulty: 2

Preferably, prepare sauce 1 day in advance
Refrigeration time of sauce before serving: 2 hours

5	VEGETABLES IN COLD OREGANO SAUCE			
	Ingredients for 2 to 4 portions	**Equivalences**		**Calories**
▪	1 cup baby carrots, raw and peeled			30.00
▪	1 cup cherry tomatoes, peeled and seeded			36.24
▪	1 cup small radishes, washed and trimmed			15.93
▪	1 cup baby corn, canned			38.00
▪	1 cup broccoli florets, blanched			27.90
		Total Calories		**148.07**

	SAUCE (1 ½ cup)			
		Equivalences		**Calories**
▪	1½ cup low fat plain yogurt			200.00
▪	1 teaspoon fresh oregano, finely chopped			0.00
▪	½ teaspoon greated lemon peal			0.00
▪	a pinch of salt and pepper			0.40
▪	¼ teaspoon splenda * or			0.00
	¼ teaspoon brown sugar *			5.00
*	optional	**Total Calories**		**205.40**

→ Cover a large colander with strong paper towel or cheese cloth. → Place colander on a bowl and pour in the yogurt. → Refrigerate for at least 2 hours, preferably overnight to drain fluid until yogurt thickens. → Discard filtered liquid and pour yogurt into a medium bowl. → Add oregano, lemon zest and sugar. → Season with salt and pepper and mix well. → Cover and refrigerate for at least 2 more hours. → Pour yogurt sauce into a small bowl just before serving. → Place vegetables on a tray, grouping them by colors or shapes, as desired. → Serve as appetizer or first course.

see blanching vegetables

6. POKER OF VEGETABLES À LA CRÈME

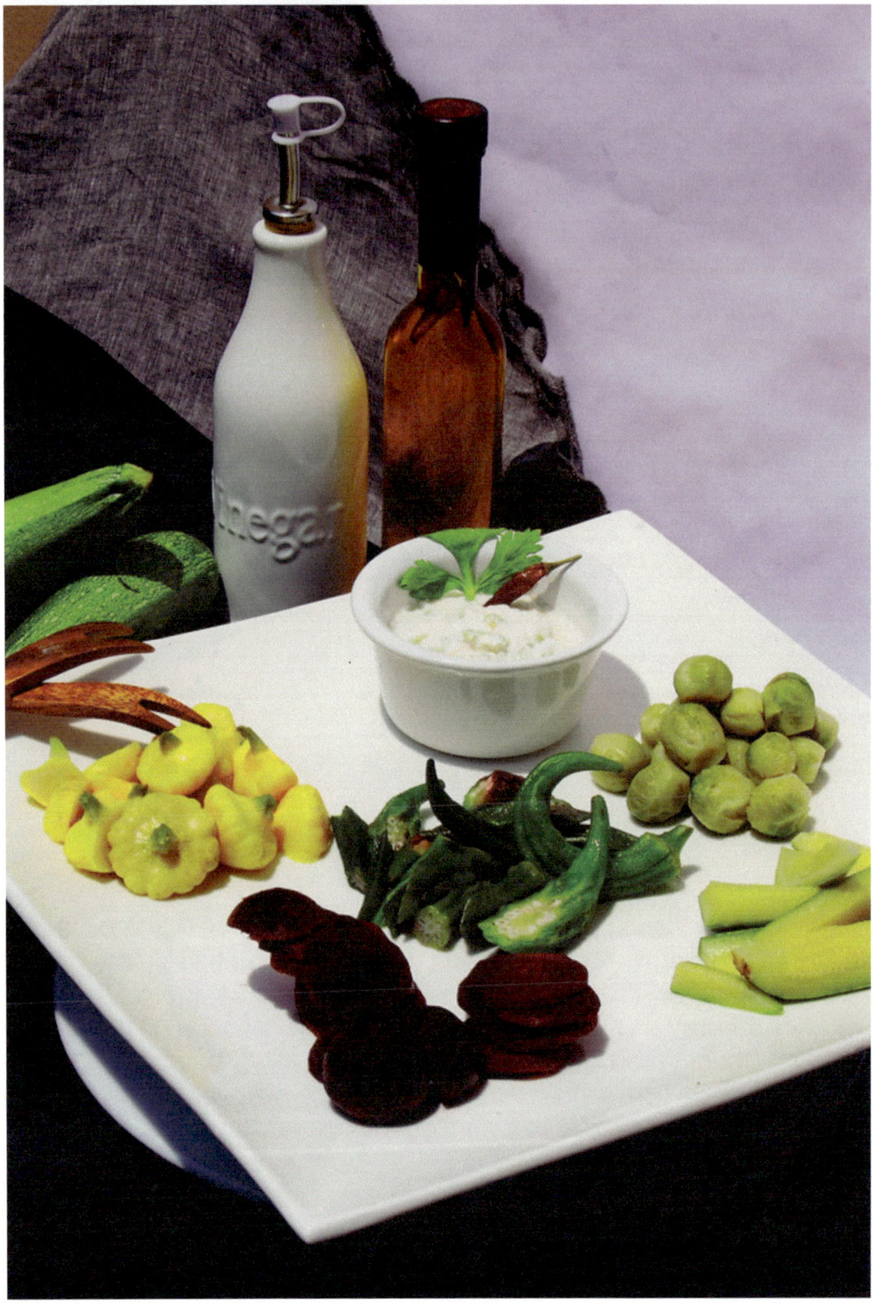

Serves 2-4
Preparation time: 30 minutes
Refrigeration time of sauce before serving: 1 hour

6	POKER OF VEGETABLES À LA CRÈME			
	Ingredients for 2 to 4 portions	**Equivalences**		**Calories**
▪	15 Brussels sprouts	1	cup	35.70
▪	15 small squashes	1	cup	27.30
▪	3 small zucchini	1	cup	60.00
▪	1 cup beet, peeled			30.10
▪	8 small okra	1	cup	50.00
		Total Calories		**203.10**

	DIPPING SAUCE (1/2 cup)			
		Equivalences		**Calories**
▪	4 tablespoons low-fat cottage cheese	½	cup	80.00
▪	2 tablespoons apple cider vinegar			1.15
▪	¼ cup finely chopped celery			6.94
▪	¼ teaspoon dried oregano			0.00
▪	a pinch of salt and pepper			0.40
▪	a pinch of Peruvian hot pepper or cayenne pepper *			0.00
*	or powdered peperoncino hot (optional)	**Total Calories**		**88.49**

→ Blanch vegetables. → Peel and cut beet into medium slices. → Slice zucchini into thick strips. → Set aside. → Mix cottage cheese, vinegar, raw chopped celery and powdered oregano until creamy. → Season with salt and pepper and carefully add cayenne pepper to taste. → Mix well and chill for 1 hour. → Place vegetables on a large plate. →. → Mix cream dipping sauce empty into a small bowl and serve with vegetables.

see blanching vegetables

7. SPINACH AND MUSHROOM SOUFFLÉ

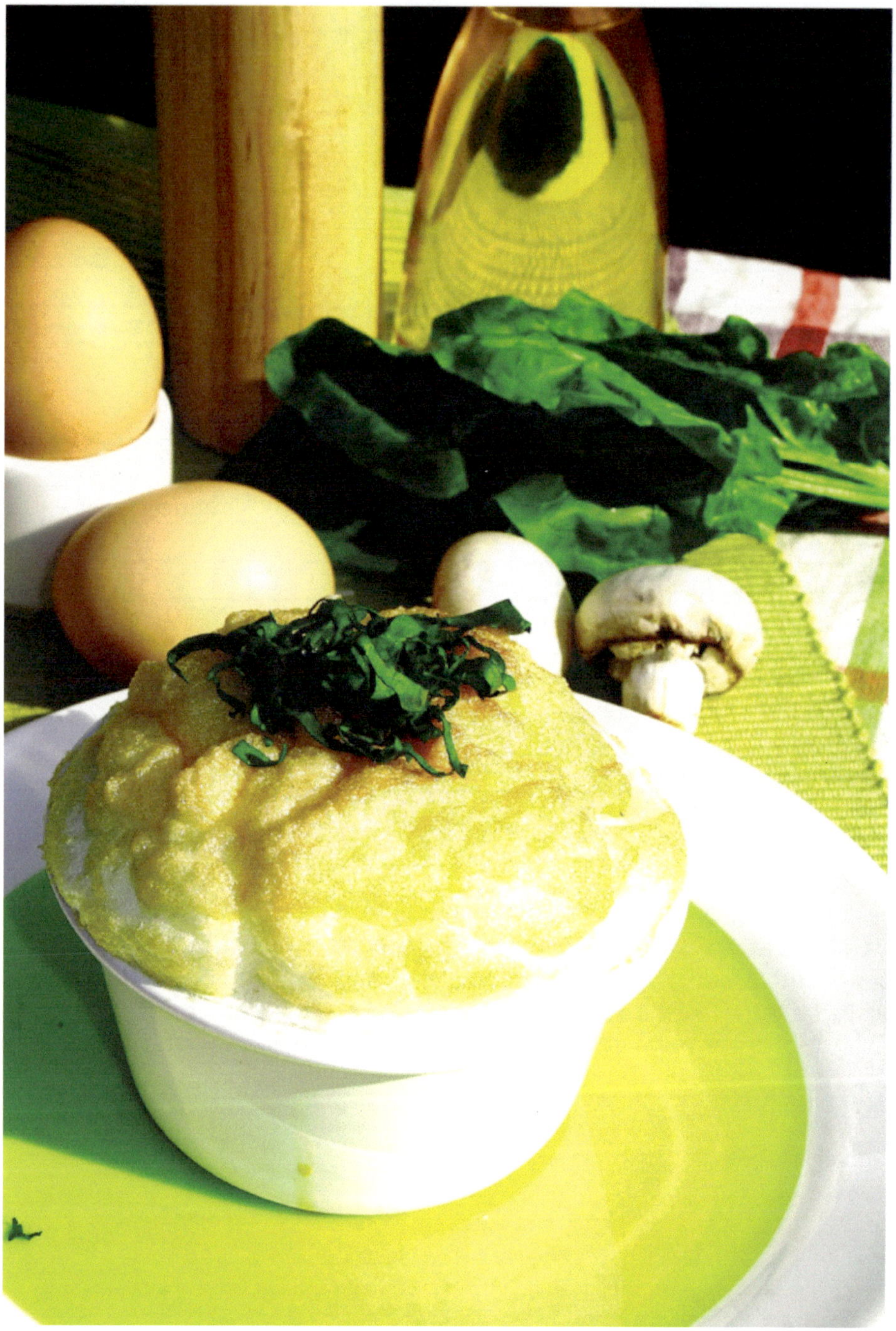

Serves 2
Preparation time: 30 minutes
Degree of difficulty: 4

7	SPINACH AND MUSHROOM SOUFFLÉ			
	Ingredients for 2 portions	**Equivalences**		**Calories**
■	1 cup fresh or defrosted spinach, chopped			4.40
■	2 eggs, preferably *Omega-3* egg			180.00
■	½ cup skim milk			50.00
■	½ cup mushrooms, sliced			4.16
■	½ cup low fat ricotta cheese, crumbled			100.00
■	¼ cup fresh parsley, chopped			0.00
■	1 tablespoon extra virgin olive or avocado oil			134.00
■	½ teaspoon butter **with salt** to grease baking pan			18.50
■	a pinch of salt and pepper			0.40
		Total Calories		**491.46**

Preheat oven to 390° F – 200° C

→ Blanch spinach and drain. → Mix in a bowl spinach, skim milk and slightly beaten egg yolks. → Set aside. → Heat oil in a non-stick frying pan. → Add sliced mushrooms and chopped parsley, and sauté for 1 minute. → Remove from heat and let it cool. → Set aside. → Use a wisk to beat egg whites in a bowl until stiff. → Add spinach and mushroom mixtures. → Mix all together with gentle folding movements, using a spatula. → Season with salt and pepper. → Grease a small baking pan with butter then empty the mixture into the pan. → Top with ricotta cheese. → Bake for approximately 12 minutes or until slightly brown. → Remove soufflé from oven and serve immediately.

* To find out if the soufflé is ready, insert a toothpick in the preparation; if it comes out clean and dry, the soufflé is ready. With practice, you may know the exact cooking time without using the toothpick. As a result, soufflé will keep its characteristic appearance and volume.

see blanching vegetables
see sautéing

SIDES

1. BROWN RICE WITH VEGETABLES

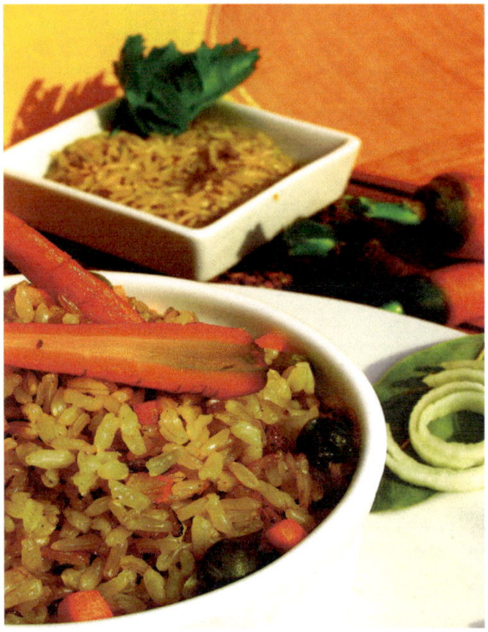

Serves 4
Preparation time: 30 minutes
Degree of difficulty: 3

1	BROWN RICE WITH VEGETABLES			
	Ingredients for 4 portions	Equivalences		Calories
▪	1 cup brown rice, quick cooking			327.00
▪	1 tablespoon extra virgin olive or avocado oil			134.00
▪	¼ cup peas			18.50
▪	¼ cup carrot, diced			7.50
▪	½ bay leaf			0.00
▪	1 small celery stalk			3.47
▪	3 slices leek			9.90
▪	2 ½ cups chicken broth or boiled water			0.00
▪	a pinch of salt			0.40
		Total Calories		**500.77**

→ Heat oil in a medium-sized pot. → Sear rice. → Gradually add **very hot** chicken broth or water and raw vegetables. → Season with salt. → Bring to a boil and stir gently with a fork. → Cover and cook over maximum heat for 5 minutes. → Reduce heat and simmer for 20 minutes or until rice is cooked. → Remove pot from heat, stir rice with a fork and let stand covered for a few minutes. → Serve warm. → We recommend ½ cup of cooked rice per person.

see searing rice

2. HOT VEGETABLES

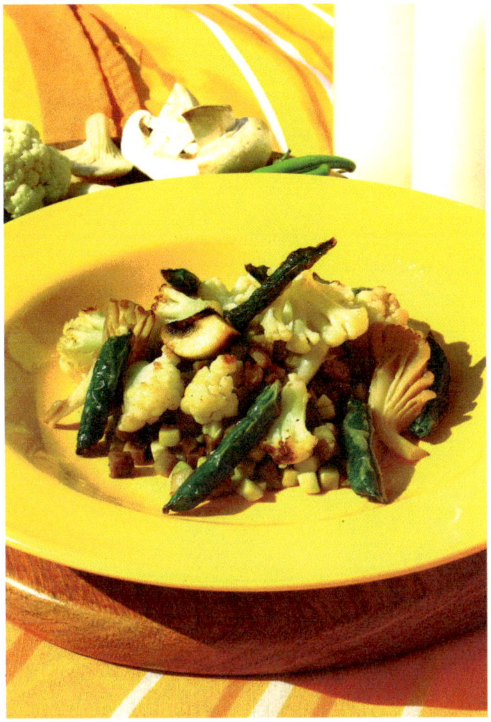

Serves 2
Preparation time: 20 minutes
Degree of difficulty: 2

2	HOT VEGETABLES			
	Ingredients for 2 portions	**Equivalences**		**Calories**
■	1 cup green beans, cut diagonally			28.60
■	½ cup fresh raw mushrooms, cut into quarters			8.98
■	½ cup eggplant, washed, unpeeled, and diced			8.28
■	½ cup zucchini, unpeeled, seeded and diced			14.08
■	½ cup cauliflower florets			11.10
■	1 tablespoon extra-virgin olive or avocado oil			134.00
■	1 tablespoon butter (optional)			111.10
■	a pinch of salt and pepper			0.40
		Total Calories		**316.54**

→ Blanch zucchini, cauliflower florets and green beans. → Set aside. → Heat oil in a non stick frying pan. → Add blanched vegetables, eggplant and mushrooms. → Sauté stirring carefully for ½ minute. → Season with salt and pepper. → Remove from heat and add melted butter. → Serve warm.

see washing eggplant
see blanching vegetables
see sautéing

3. BAKED OR GRILLED POTATO

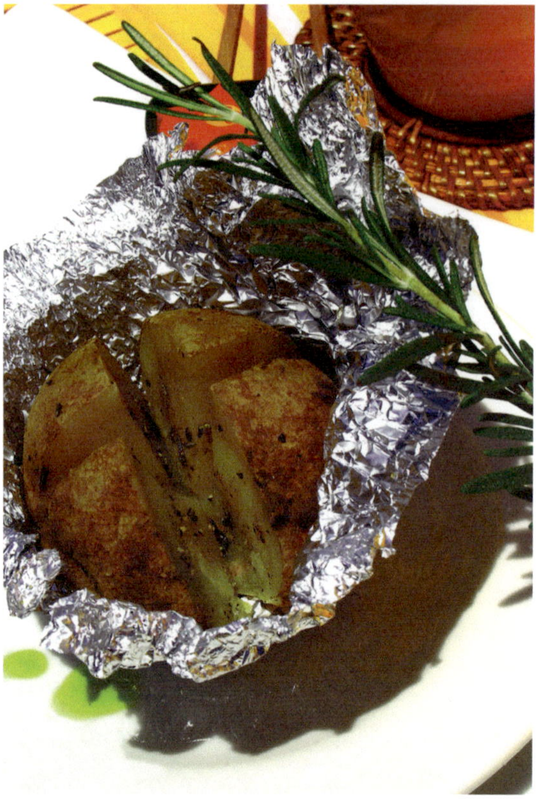

Serves 2
Preparation time: 50 minutes
Degree of difficulty: 1

3	BAKED OR GRILLED POTATO			
	Ingredients for 2 portions	**Equivalences**		**Calories**
▪	1 medium sized potato, with skin			72.27
▪	a pinch of dried rosemary			0.00
▪	a pinch of salt and pepper			0.40
▪	aluminum foil			–
		Total Calories		**72.67**

Preheat oven: 390° F – 200° C

→ Wash potato and dry well, leaving skin on. → Cross-cut potato and season with salt, pepper and powdered rosemary. → Wrap potato in aluminum foil. → Place in oven (or on grill) for approximately 45 minutes or until cooked. → Remove from oven or grill. → Discard aluminum wrap. → Serve half a potato per person.

4. SMALL POTATOES WITH PARSLEY

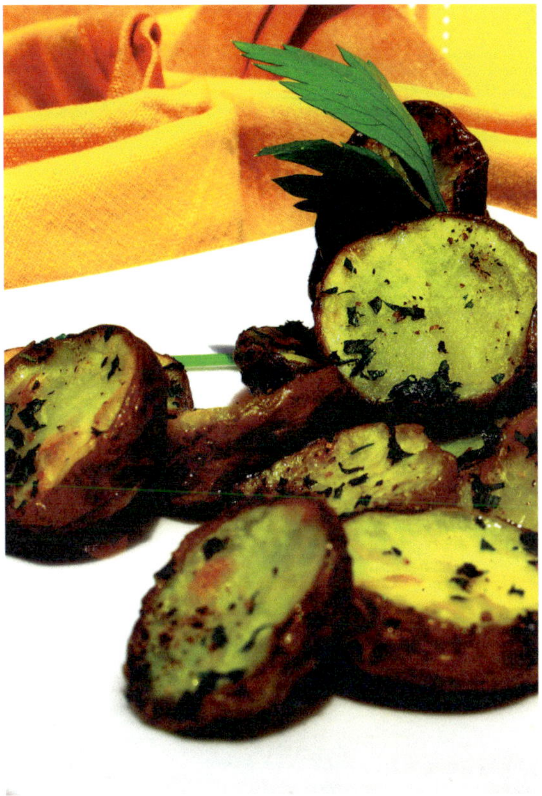

Serves 2
Preparation time: 12 minutes
Degree of difficulty: 2

4	SMALL POTATOES WITH PARSLEY			
	Ingredients for 2 portions	**Equivalences**		**Calories**
▪	10 small potatoes with skin			72.27
▪	1 teaspoon fresh parsley, chopped			0.00
▪	1 clove garlic			5.70
▪	1 tablespoon extra-virgin olive or avocado oil			134.00
▪	½ tablespoon unsalted butter			55.55
▪	a pinch of salt and pepper			0.40
		Total Calories		**267.92**

→ Wash potatoes well, leaving skin on. → Place in pot of boiling water to cover. → Cook for approximately 10 minutes until they are nearly done. → Remove potatoes from heat and drain. → Cut some potatoes into halves, and some others into fourths. → Set aside. → Heat oil in a non-stick frying pan. → Add garlic. → Fry and brown evenly. → Discard garlic. → Add potatoes and chopped parsley. → Season with salt and pepper. → Sauté for a few minutes until crispy and golden. → Serve warm.

see frying
see sautéing

5. SMALL BAKED POTATOES WITH OLIVE OIL

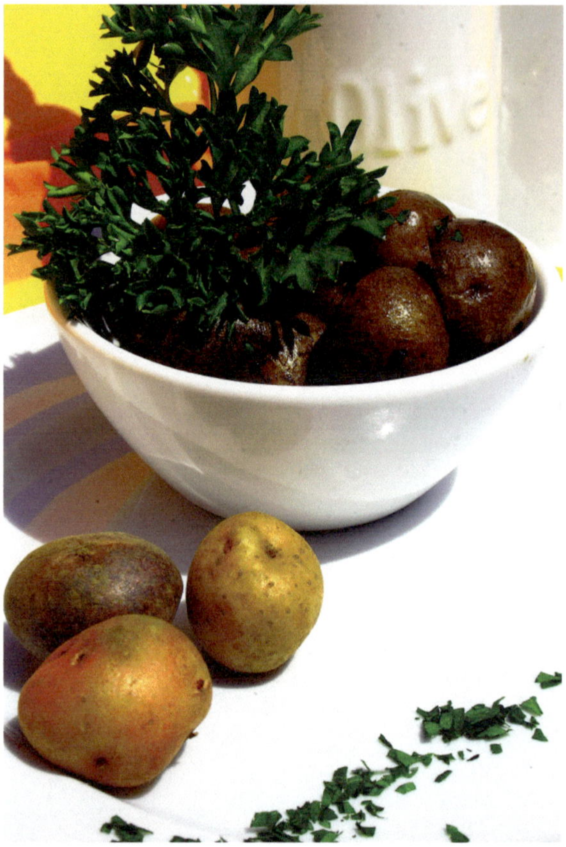

Serves 2
Preparation time: 20 minutes
Degree of difficulty: 2

5	SMALL BAKED POTATOES WITH OLIVE OIL			
	Ingredients for 2 portions	**Equivalences**		**Calories**
▪	10 small potatoes, with skin			72.27
▪	1 tablespoon extra virgin olive or avocado oil			134.00
▪	1 teaspoon fresh coriander, coarsely chopped or pinched dried			0.00
▪	1 teaspoon fresh thyme or pinch of dried thyme			0.00
▪	a pinch of salt and pepper			0.40
		Total Calories		**206.67**

Preheat oven to 390º F – 200º C

→ Wash potatoes well leaving skin on. → Place them in pot of boiling water. → Cook for approximately 8 minutes. → Remove when nearly done and drain in colander. → Place on a baking dish and sprinkle with oil. → Mix with coriander and thyme. → Season with salt and pepper. → Bake for 15 minutes until potatoes are cooked and crispy. → Serve immediately.

6. SPINACH PURÉE

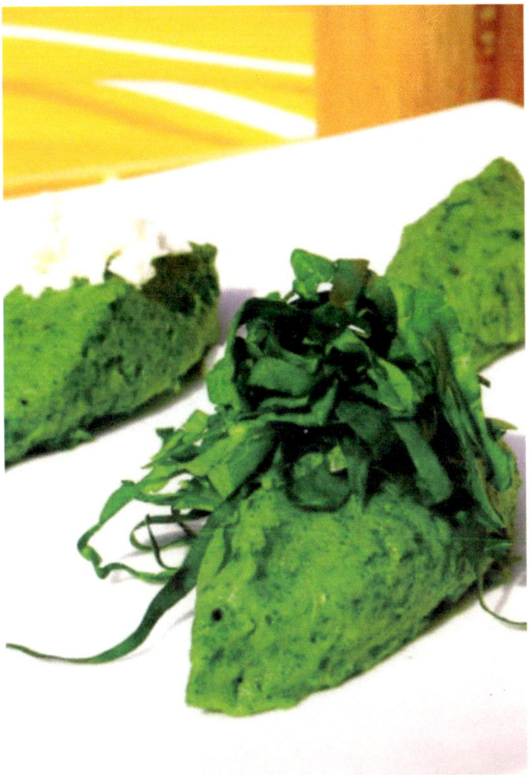

Serves 2
Preparation time: 20 minutes
Degree of difficulty: 2

6	SPINACH PURÉE			
	Ingredients for 2 portions	Equivalences		Calories
▪	2 cups fresh or defrosted spinach leaves			8.80
▪	1 medium sized yellow or white potato, whole			72.27
▪	¼ cup low fat feta cheese			40.00
▪	1 tablespoon skim milk			10.00
▪	¼ teaspoon dried nutmeg			0.00
▪	a pinch of salt and pepper			0.40
		Total Calories		**131.47**

→ Boil whole potato. → Remove from heat and drain. → While still warm, peel potato carefully and press with fork, until pureed. → Set aside. → Blanch spinach leaves. → Dry spinach and blend with cheese and milk. → Empty ingredients into a medium-sized pot. → Heat over a low flame for 3 minutes, constantly stirring. → Add pureed potato and nutmeg. → Season with salt and pepper and mix well. → Remove pan from heat. → If you want it to be a creamier and lump free purée, strain. → Serve warm.

see blanching vegetables

7. COUNTRY-STYLE MASHED POTATOES

Chef Marcelo Portuondo's recipe

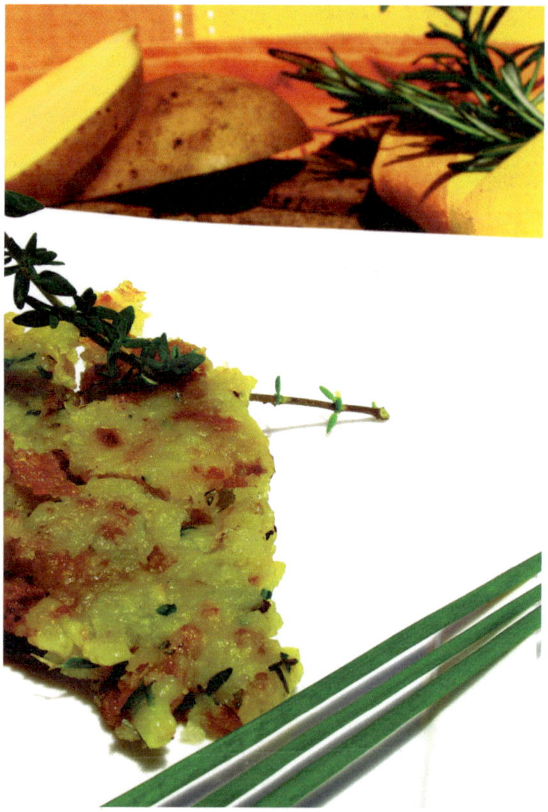

Serves 2
Preparation time: 30 minutes
Degree of difficulty: 2

7	COUNTRY-STYLE MASHED POTATOES			
	Ingredients for 2 portions	Equivalences		Calories
▪	2 medium sized potatoes			144.54
▪	¼ teaspoon dried rosemary			0.00
▪	¼ teaspoon dried thyme			0.00
▪	¼ teaspoon chives, finely chopped			0.00
▪	1 tablespoon garlic oil			139.70
▪	a pinch of salt and pepper			0.40
		Total Calories		**284.64**

Preheat oven: 390º F – 200º C

→ Boil potatoes. → Remove from heat and drain. → When still hot, sleep off the potatoes skin and press with a fork to purée. → Season with salt and pepper. → Add warm garlic oil, rosemary, thyme and chives to mashed potatoes. → Mix well. → Place in baking dish. Bake for 20 minutes, or until golden and surface has formed a thin crust. → Serve warm.

see garlic oil

8. GLAZED CARROTS

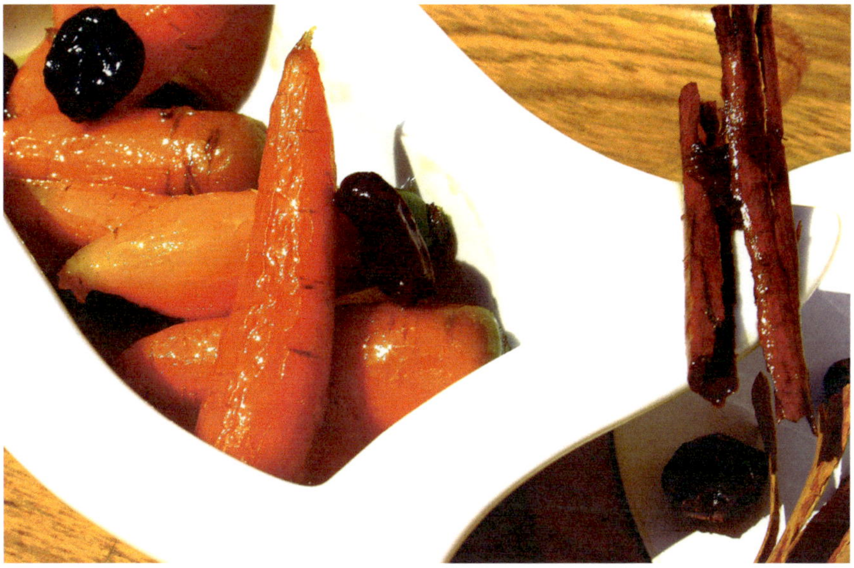

Serves 2
Preparation time: 20 minutes
Degree of difficulty: 2

8	GLAZED CARROTS			
	Ingredients for 2 portions	Equivalences		Calories
▪	2 cups raw baby carrots			60.00
▪	½ cup splenda or			0.00
	3 tablespoon brown sugar			60.00
▪	½ cup water			0.00
▪	2 cinnamon sticks			0.00
▪	10 brown raisins			26.00
▪	½ tablespoon butter			55.55
		Total Calories		**201.55**

→ Place washed carrots in a small pot and cover with water. → Add sugar and cinnamon sticks. → Stir with a wooden spoon. → Cover and cook over a low flame for 10 minutes. → Add raisins and cook for 10 more minutes or until carrots are tender, avoiding boiling it dry → Remove from heat, discard cinnamon and add melted butter. → Mix and serve warm.

SALADS

1. CABBAGE, CARROT AND RAISIN CHINESE SALAD

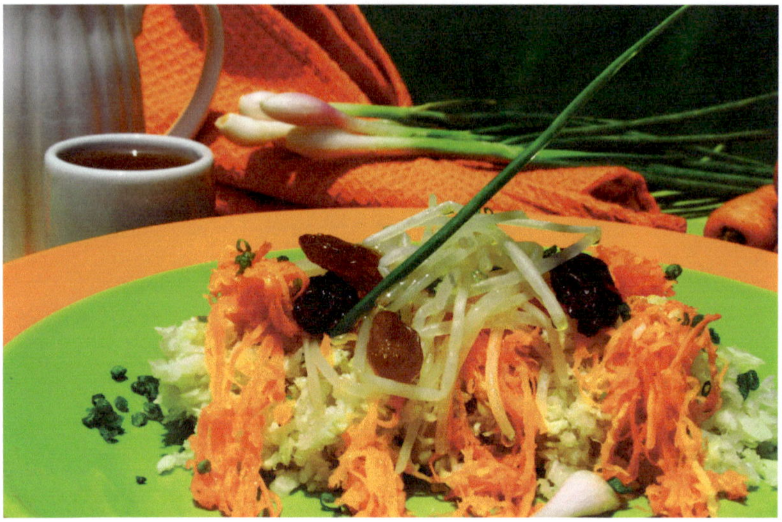

Serves 2
Preparation time: 10 minutes
Degree of difficulty: 2

1	CABBAGE, CARROT AND RAISIN CHINESE SALAD			
	Ingredients for 2 portions	**Equivalences**		**Calories**
▪	1 cup mung bean sprouts			14.40
▪	1 cup white cabbage, finely shredded			24.50
▪	½ cup carrots, finely shredded *			15.00
▪	¼ cup scallions, finely chopped			5.00
▪	10 golden or brown raisins			26.00
▪	¼ teaspoon splenda (optional) or			0.00
	¼ teaspoon brown sugar (optional)			5.00
▪	4 tablespoons *sweet and sour vinaigrette*			52.30
▪	a pinch of salt and pepper			0.40
	* drain water excess with paper towel	**Total Calories**		**142.60**

→ Blanch mung bean sprouts. → Wrap in paper towel and dry well. → Place in a salad bowl and mix with shredded cabbage. → Add shredded carrots, finely chopped scallions and raisins. → Bring it all together and add *sweet and sour vinaigrette*. → Serve immediately.

see Sweet and Sour Vinaigrette
see blanching vegetables

2. OLIVE, PEPPER AND COTTAGE CHEESE SALAD

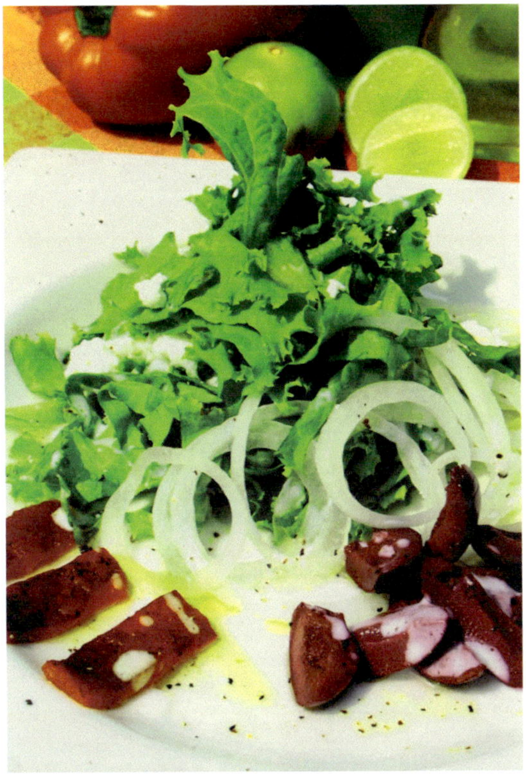

Serves 2
Preparation time: 10 minutes
Degree of difficulty: 2

2	OLIVE, PEPPER AND COTTAGE CHEESE SALAD			
	Ingredients for 2 portions	Equivalences		Calories
▪	6 leaves romaine lettuce, chopped into thin strips	¾	cup	8.32
▪	½ cup red peppers, lightly roasted and chopped into thick strips			10.40
▪	1 medium sized white onion, cut into thin rings	½	cup	8.15
▪	½ cup low fat cottage cheese			80.00
▪	½ cup low fat plain yogurt			80.00
▪	10 black seedless olives	¼	cup	216.80
▪	1 tablespoon extra virgin olive or avocado oil *			134.00
▪	½ tablespoon lemon juice, to taste			0.80
▪	a pinch of salt and pepper			0.40
*	or any other gourmet oil of your choice	Total Calories		**538.87**

→ Wash and chop lettuce leaves. → Dry well and set aside. → Cut onion into thin rings. → Wash onions in a bowl with water and a pinch of salt. → Drain well in a colander and set aside. → Halve the olives. → Set aside. → Place lettuce leaves, onion rings, peppers and olives in a salad bowl. → Mix together with cheese. → Dress with oil and lemon juice before serving. → Season with salt and pepper. → Dress the salad with chilled beaten yogurt. → Serve immediately.

see slightly roasting peppers

3. EGGPLANT, PEPPER AND ROSEMARY SALAD

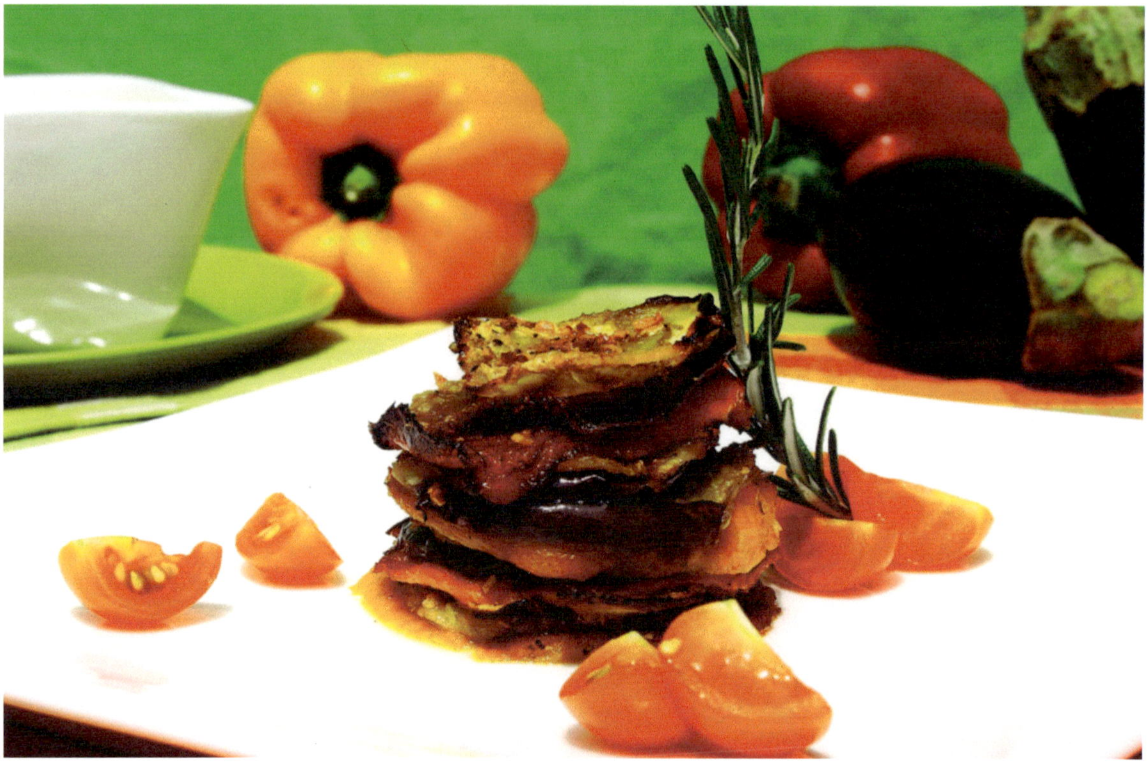

Serves 2
Preparation time: 20-30 minutes
Degree of difficulty: 3

3	EGGPLANT, PEPPER AND ROSEMARY SALAD			
	Ingredients for 2 portions	**Equivalences**		**Calories**
▪	1 red pepper, lightly roasted and cut into rectangles	1	cup	20.80
▪	1 yellow pepper, lightly roasted and cut into rectangles	1	cup	20.80
▪	2 medium sized eggplants, unpeeled	2	cups	33.12
▪	1 cup cherry tomatoes peeled, seeded and cut into quarters			27.40
▪	1 clove garlic, sliced	¼	tbs.	4.60
▪	2 sprigs fresh rosemary			0.00
▪	1 tablespoon extra virgin olive oil, for baking			134.00
▪	1 tablespoon extra virgin olive oil, for dressing			134.00
▪	¼ tablespoon balsamic vinegar, for dressing			6.00
▪	a pinch of salt and pepper			0.40
		Total Calories		**381.12**

Preheat oven: 320º F – 160º C

→ Cut eggplants into medium slices. → Wash and drain. → Place eggplants and peppers on a baking dish. → Top with rosemary springs and sliced garlic. → Spray with virgin olive oil and season with salt and pepper. → Bake in oven for approximately 30 minutes or until golden. → Remove from oven and let cool. → Place baked eggplants on a shallow salad plate, alternating with peppers. → Garnish with quartered tomatoes. → Dress with extra-virgin olive oil, balsamic vinegar, salt and pepper. → Serve immediately.

Note: Eggplants and peppers will be crispy if the oven is preheated to 390ºF, and they are baked for only 15 minutes. **We recommend you carefully watch the cooking process to avoid burning them.**

see slightly roasting peppers

see washing eggplants

see peeling raw tomatoes

4. ASPARAGUS AND BROCCOLI SALAD

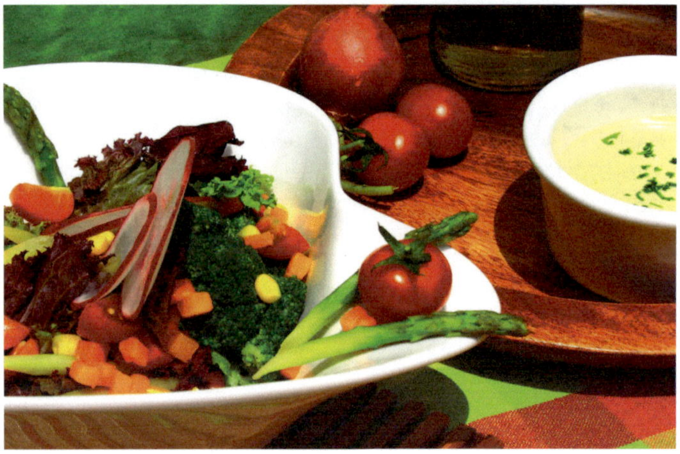

Serves 2
Preparation time: 15-20 minutes
Degree of difficulty: 2

4	ASPARAGUS AND BROCCOLI SALAD			
	Ingredients for 2 portions	**Equivalences**		**Calories**
▪	1 cup asparagus cut into thirds, snap off tough ends			17.97
▪	1 cup broccoli florets			27.90
▪	½ cup radishes, washed and finely sliced			8.00
▪	½ cup cherry tomatoes, peeled and seeded			18.12
▪	8 leaves green and red lettuce, washed			10.00
▪	¼ cup canned and drained corn			285.00
▪	½ cup carrots, finely diced			19.00
▪	2 tablespoons *Homemade Mayonnaise*			254.70
▪	¼ teaspoon fresh parsley, chopped			0.60
▪	a pinch of salt and pepper			0.40
		Total Calories		**641.69**

→ Cut and blanch asparagus, broccoli and carrots. → Let cool and set aside. → Place lettuce leaves in a deep salad bowl. → Add cold blanched vegetables, tomatoes and drained corn over the lettuce. → Add sliced radishes. → Mix chopped parsley with *Homemade Mayonnaise*. → Pour dressing over salad just before serving.

see Homemade Mayonnaise
see blanching vegetables
see peeling raw tomatoes

5. BABY SPINACH SALAD

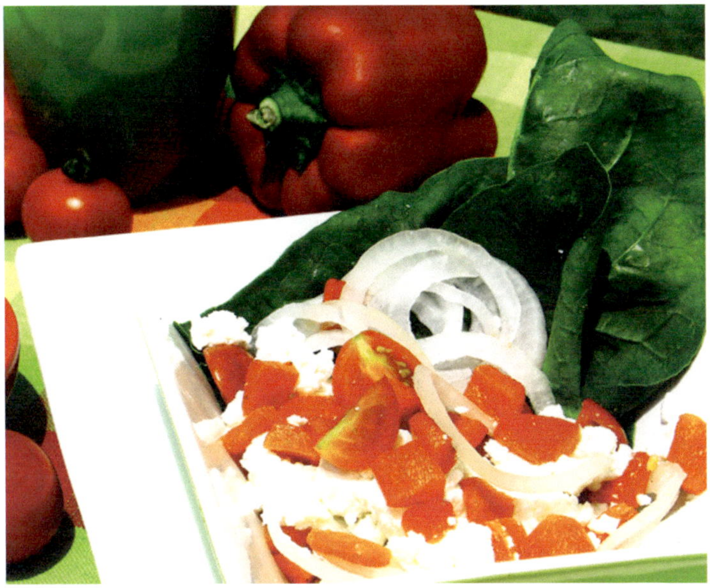

Serves 2
Preparation time: 20 minutes
Degree of difficulty: 2

5	BABY SPINACH SALAD			
	Ingredients for 2 portions	**Equivalences**		**Calories**
▪	2 cups baby spinach leaves, washed well			8.80
▪	1 cup white onion, cut into thin rings			16.30
▪	½ cup lightly roasted red pepper, cut into small cubes	½	cup	10.40
▪	¼ cup low fat feta cheese, crumbled			40.00
▪	¼ cup low fat cottage cheese			50.00
▪	1 cherry tomato for garnish			4.00
▪	2 tablespoons *Mustard Vinaigrette*			96.81
		Total Calories		**226.31**

→ Wash onion rings in a bowl with water and a pinch of salt. → Drain well in colander. → Set aside. → Place drained spinach leaves in a deep salad bowl. → Mix with onion rings and roasted peppers. → Combine cheeses and add to bowl. → Mix gently. → Garnish with a cherry tomato. → Add *Mustard Vinaigrette* to salad just before serving.

see slightly roasting peppers
see Mustard Vinaigrette

6. SPINACH AND MUSHROOM SALAD IN SOY SAUCE

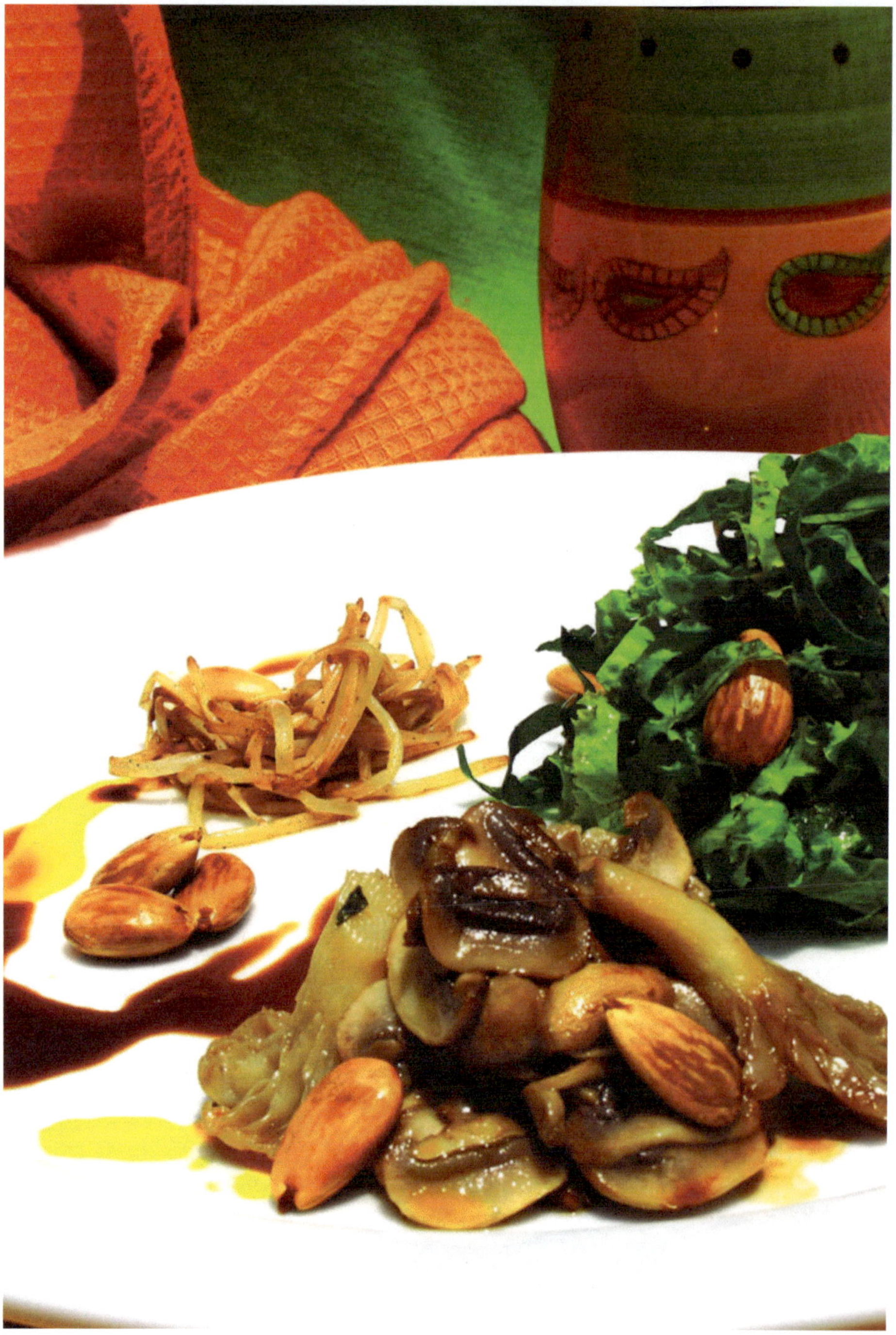

Serves 2
Preparation time: 15 minutes
Degree of difficulty: 3

6	SPINACH AND MUSHROOM SALAD IN SOY SAUCE			
	Ingredients for 2 portions	**Equivalences**		**Calories**
■	2 cups fresh spinach			8.80
■	1 ½ cups lettuce (any type)			16.64
■	1 cup raw mushrooms, whole or sliced			17.96
■	½ cup blanched mung bean sprouts			7.20
■	10 toasted almonds			62.14
■	½ tablespoon balsamic vinegar			6.00
■	1 tablespoon low sodium soy sauce			10.00
■	1 tablespoon extra-virgin olive or avocado oil *			134.00
■	a pinch of salt and pepper			0.40
*	or any other gourmet oil of your choice	**Total Calories**		**263.14**

→ Separate oil into three equal parts. → Wash lettuce, tear apart by hand and dry well. → Place in a deep salad bowl. → Wash mushrooms, then cut and set aside. → Wash spinach and cut it into thin strips. → Dry with paper towel and set aside. → Place one third tablespoon of oil in a deep frying pan or wok, over a high heat. → Add spinach and sauté very lightly turning with tongs until liquid evaporates. → Set aside. → Place lettuce leaves in a deep salad bowl. → Arrange spinach over lettuce. → Add one third of oil to the frying pan and sauté mushrooms for 2 minutes. → Remove from heat and sprinkle over spinach. → In the frying pan add remaining ingredients: oil, soy sauce and vinegar. → Add blanched mung bean sprouts and lightly sauté. → Season with salt and pepper. → As soon it begins to boil, remove from heat and add hot sprouts to salad. → Garnish with toasted almonds. → Serve warm and eat immediately so vegetables will not wilt.

see blanching vegetables
see toasting almonds
see sautéing

7. CHICKPEAS AND SPROUT SALAD

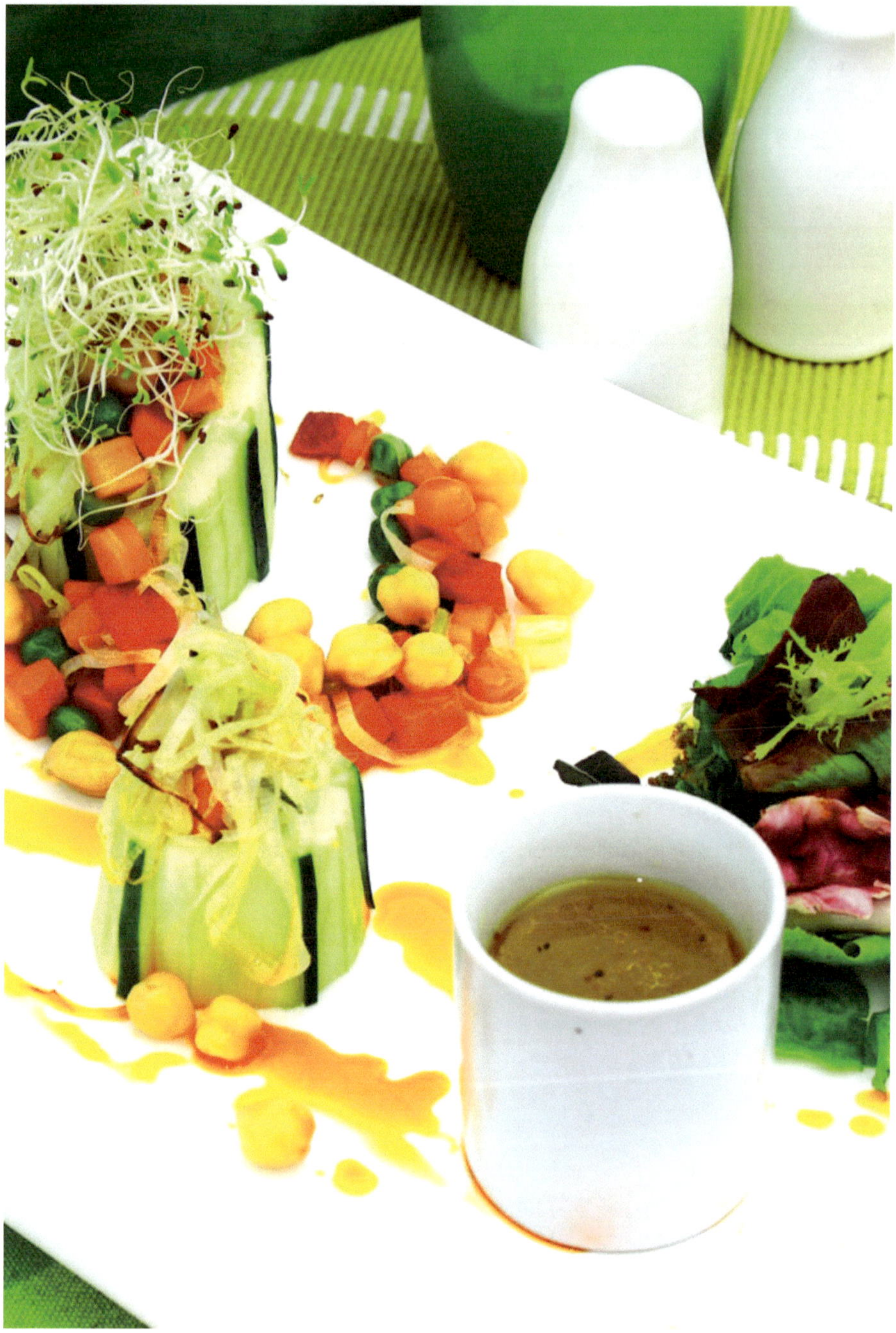

Serves 2
Preparation time: 30 minutes
Degree of difficulty: 3

7	CHICK-PEAS AND SPROUT SALAD			
	Ingredients for 2 portions	**Equivalences**		**Calories**
▪	½ cup whole chickpeas			340.80
▪	6 lettuce leaves, cut into pieces	2	cups	10.00
▪	¼ cup leek, sliced into thin rings			7.15
▪	¼ cup green peas			30.00
▪	¼ cup carrots, cut into small cubes			9.50
▪	¼ cup peeled cucumbers, cut into small cubes			5.00
▪	a handful of alfalfa sprouts, rinsed	1	cup	6.00
▪	1 dry bay leaf			0.00
▪	1 tablespoon extra virgin olive or avocado oil *			134.00
▪	4 tablespoons *Lemon Dressing* or the amount desired			90.80
*	or any other gourmet oil of your choice	**Total Calories**		**633.25**

→ Cook chickpeas in advance, or use canned. → Allow to cool. → Set aside. → Blanch peas, peppers, and carrots. → Set aside. → Heat oil in a deep non stick pan, and sauté leek, peppers, peas and carrots. → Allow to cool, then add cucumber. → Arrange lettuce pieces in a salad dish. → Add cold vegetables on top of lettuce. → Add cold chickpeas and cover with alfalfa sprouts. → Dress before serving.

Note: → For the artistic presentation of this recipe, use a potato peeler to shave off most of the skin going from one end to the other. → Slice into 3-4 very thick sections. → Core the sections of seeds and much of the pulp. → Use hollow sections on end to fill with the ingredients above.

see Lemon Dressing
see washing and cooking legumes al dente
see blanching vegetables
see sautéing

8. HEART OF PALM AND SUN-DRIED TOMATO SALAD

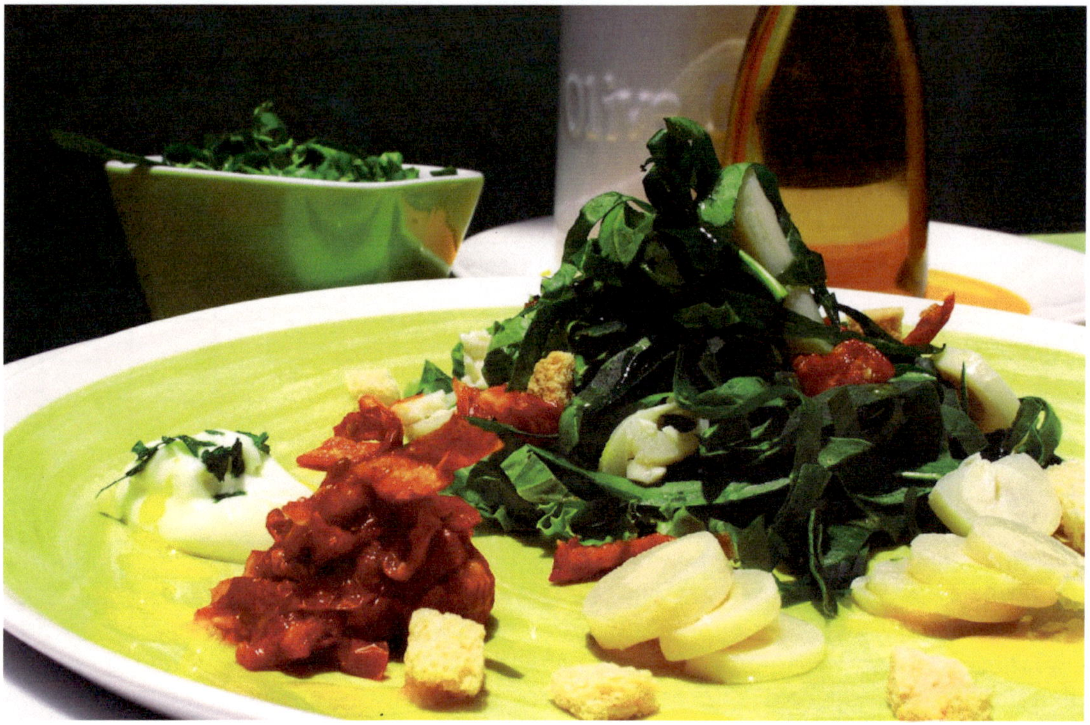

Serves 2
Preparation time: 10 minutes
Degree of difficulty: 2

8	HEART OF PALM AND SUNDRIED TOMATO SALAD			
	Ingredients for 2 portions	Equivalences		Calories
▪	4 leaves lettuce, washed and cut into strips	½	cup	5.00
▪	8 leaves fresh spinach, washed and cut into strips	1	cup	5.70
▪	6 slices sundried tomatoes			1.09
▪	4 stalks of hearts of palm, packed in water	1	cup	39.00
▪	2 tablespoons *Homemade Mayonnaise*			254.70
▪	¼ cup whole wheat bread croutons (optional)			36.50
		Total Calories		**341.99**

→ Soak died tomatoes in warm water for 10 minutes. → Drain water excess. → Cut into thin strips. → Set aside. → Combine lettuce and spinach strips in a bowl. → Add tomato slices and mix. → Cut hearts of palm into slices just before serving and place over salad. → Dress salad with *Homemade mayonnaise* and serve. → If you wish, add ¼ cup of whole wheat croutons.

see Homemade Mayonnaise
see hydrating sundried tomatoes

9. AVOCADO, LETTUCE AND TOMATO SALAD

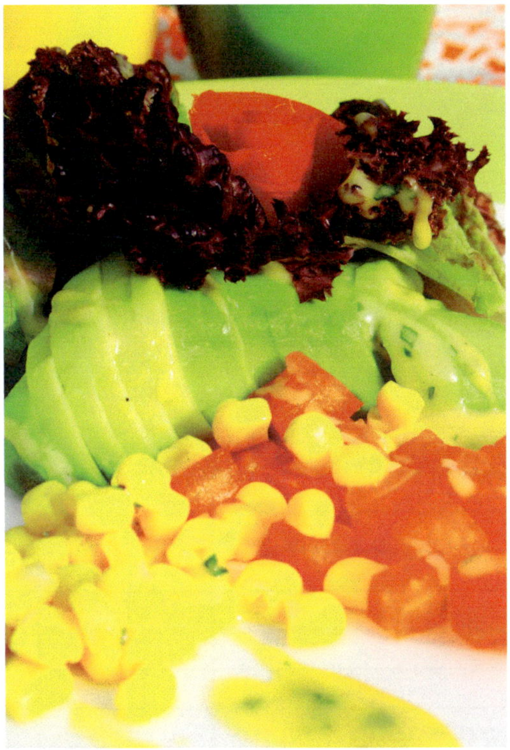

Serves 2
Preparation time: 10 minutes
Degree of difficulty: 1

9	AVOCADO, LETTUCE AND TOMATO SALAD			
	Ingredients for 2 portions	**Equivalences**		**Calories**
▪	½ ripe medium sized avocado, cut into slices[1]	¾	cup	142.00
▪	1 tablespoons lime juice, or the amount you wish			1.60
▪	2 small tomatoes, peeled, seeded, cut into medium-sized pieces	1	cup	27.50
▪	6 leaves of mixed lettuce, chopped	¾	cup	8.32
▪	¼ cup canned and drained corn			285.00
▪	2 tablespoons *Mustard Vinaigrette*			96.81
		Total Calories		**561.23**

[1] If you wish to prepare avocado beforehand, it is best to drizzle with key lime juice to prevent oxidation.

Place lettuce, tomatoes and corn in distinct piles on individual plates. → Do not mix.→ Place avocado next to the other ingredients and drizzle with *Mustard Vinaigrette*. → Serve immediately.

see peeling raw tomatoes
see Mustard Vinaigrette

Note: This salad is similar in presentation of a Cobb Salad.

10. CHICKEN, ASPARAGUS AND APPLE SALAD

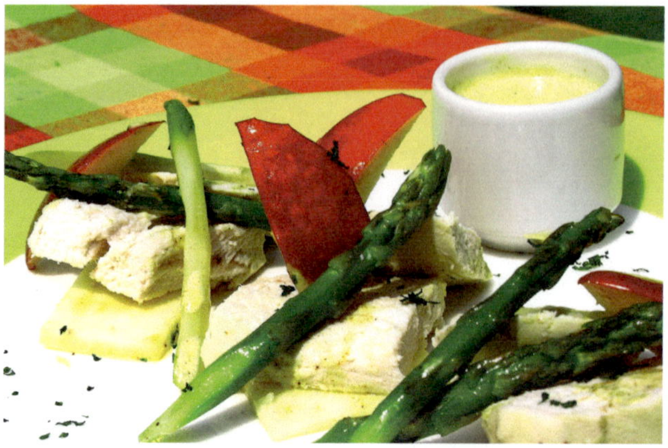

Serves 4
Preparation time: 30 minutes
Degree of difficulty: 2

10	CHICKEN, ASPARAGUS AND APPLE SALAD			
	Ingredients for 4 portions	**Equivalences**		**Calories**
▪	1 medium chicken breast, boneless and skinless (1½ cup)	360 g	0.79 lb	4.84
▪	½ medium celery stalk, cut into 1 inch	¼	cup	3.42
▪	½ medium leek, cut into 1 inch	¼	cup	9.90
▪	1 dry bay leaf			0.00
▪	2 medium red apples washed, cut into wedges	1	cup	91.96
▪	1 cup fresh or canned green asparagus, snap off ends of fresh			13.70
▪	3 tablespoons *Homemade Curried Mayonnaise*			382.05
▪	2 ½ cups water (for broth)			0.00
▪	fresh parsley, chopped, the amount optional			0.00
▪	a pinch of salt			0.40
		Total Calories		**506.27**

→ Wash chicken breast. → Heat water in a pot and add salt, celery, leek and 1 bay leaf. → Drop in chicken breast and cook for 20 minutes or until thoroughly cooked. → Remove pot from heat and allow to cool. → Cut chicken breast into medium sized bites. → Set aside. → Cut asparagus diagonally in half. → Set aside. → Core and cut unpeeled apples into wedges. → Mix ingredients together in a bowl. → Dress salad with *Homemade Curried Mayonnaise*. → Sprinkle with chopped parsley. → Serve.

Note: We suggest using the chicken broth for another recipe or adding ¼ cup of noodles to make a soup. → The remaining broth may be frozen in an airtight container for up to 1 year.

see blanching vegetables
see Homemade Curried Mayonnaise

11. CHERRY TOMATO AND NUT SALAD

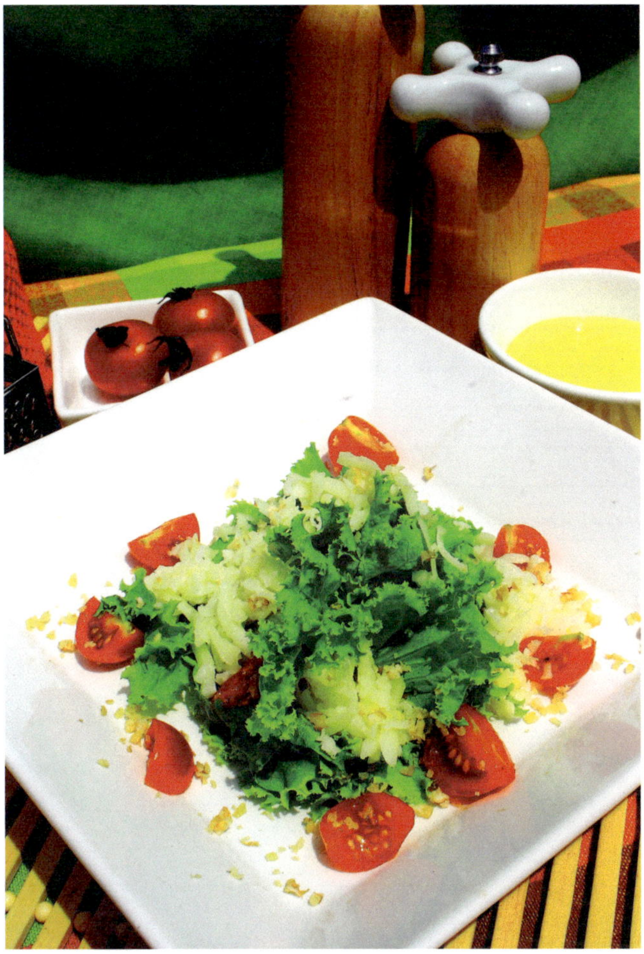

Serves 2
Preparation time: 10 minutes
Degree of difficulty: 1

11	CHERRY TOMATO AND NUT SALAD			
	Ingredients for 2 portions	**Equivalences**		**Calories**
■	1 cup cherry tomatoes, peeled and seeded, cut into half			18.12
■	6 leaves green leafy lettuce, cut into pieces	¾	cup	8.32
■	½ cup low fat, fresh mozzarella cheese, shredded in thick strips			45.00
■	8 walnuts, finely chopped			108.36
■	2 tablespoons *Homemade Mayonnaise*			254.70
		Total Calories		**434.50**

→ Wash lettuce, then drain and cut into pieces. → Place lettuce and tomatoes in a salad bowl. → Cover with shredded mozzarella cheese. → Dress the salad with *Homemade Mayonnaise*. → Garnish with chopped walnuts just before serving.

see peeling raw tomatoes
see Homemade Mayonnaise

12. *MIXED VEGETABLES WITH FETA AND PECANS*

Serves 2
Preparation time: 6 minutes
Degree of difficulty: 1

12	MIXED GREEN VEGETABLE, FETA CHEESE AND PECAN			
	Ingredients for 2 portions	**Equivalences**		**Calories**
■	8 leaves green and red lettuce, chopped	1	cup	10.00
■	¼ cup whole wheat croutons			36.50
■	5 chopped pecans	¼	cup	124.60
■	¼ cup crumbled low fat feta cheese			80.00
■	2 tablespoons *Lemon Dressing*			45.40
		Total Calories		**296.50**

→ Wash and drain well lettuce leaves, then place in a salad bowl. → Add feta cheese and pecans. → Drizzle with *Lemon Dressing* and top with croutons just before serving.

see Lemon Dressing

SOUPS AND CRÈMES

***Chef's suggestion:** Season the soups with salt and pepper at the end of the cooking process, to keep the natural flavor of the ingredients.*

1. CHICKEN BREAST BROTH

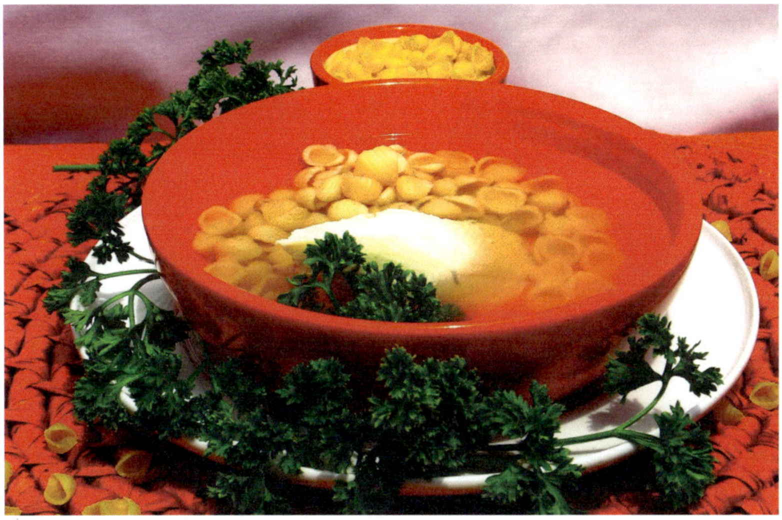

Serves 2
Preparation time: 20 minutes
Degree of difficulty: 1

1	CHICKEN BREAST BROTH			
	Ingredients for 2 portions	**Equivalences**		**Calories**
▪	1 medium sized chicken breast, bone in (1½ cup)	360 g	0.79 lb	484.00
▪	½ medium sized celery stalk, cut into large pieces	¼	cup	6.94
▪	½ medium sized leek, cut into large pieces	¼	cup	19.80
▪	1 bay leaf			0.00
▪	2 cups water			0.00
▪	½ cup noodles (optional)			171.00
▪	a pinch of salt and pepper			0.40
		Total Calories		**682.14**

→ Wash chicken breast, removing skin. → Boil water in a large pad, then add celery, leek and bay leaf. → Place chicken breast and simmer for 20 minutes, until chicken is done. → Season with salt and pepper. → Discard celery and leek. → Cut chicken breast into pieces. → Discard the bones. → Garnish with fresh parsley. → Serve warm.

Optional: → Add ½ cup of noodles and boil following directions on the package.

2. CREAM OF MUSHROOM SOUP

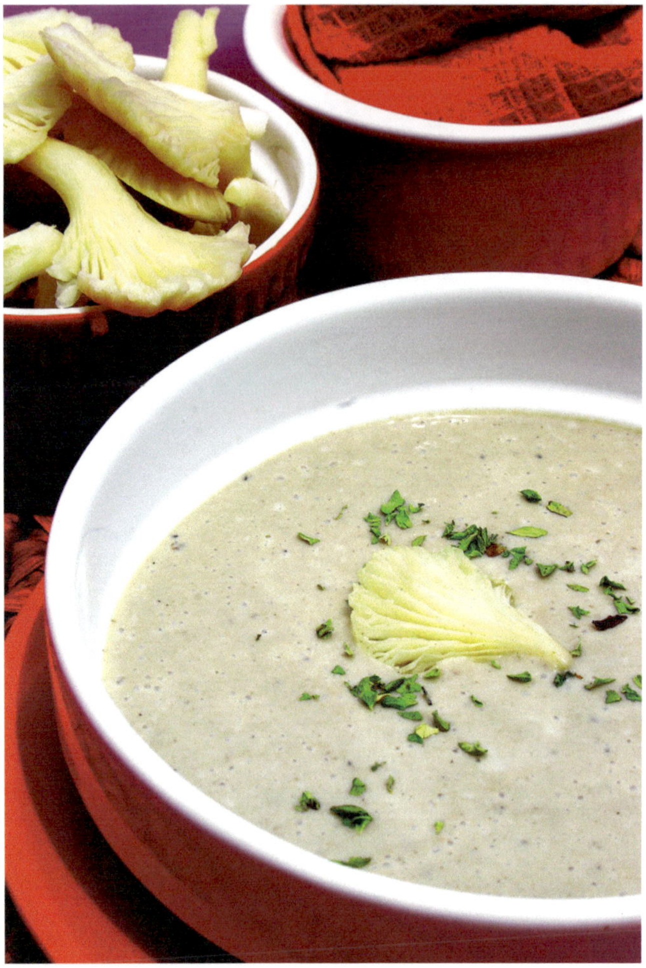

Serves 2
Preparation time: 20 minutes
Degree of difficulty: 1

2	CREAM OF MUSHROOM SOUP			
	Ingredients for 2 portions	**Equivalences**		**Calories**
▪	2 cups mushrooms, chopped			35.92
▪	½ cup skim milk			50.00
▪	2 cups water			0.00
▪	1 teaspoon parsley, finely chopped for garnishing			0.00
▪	a pinch of salt and pepper			0.40
		Total Calories		**86.32**

→ Blend mushrooms with water and simmer in a medium sized pan over low heat. → Stir with a wooden spoon. → Continue cooking for approximately 15 minutes, until liquid is reduced by half. → Season with salt and pepper. → Remove from heat and add warm milk. → Add salt to taste. → Garnish with finely chopped parsley. → Serve warm.

3. CREAM OF MIXED VEGETABLE SOUP

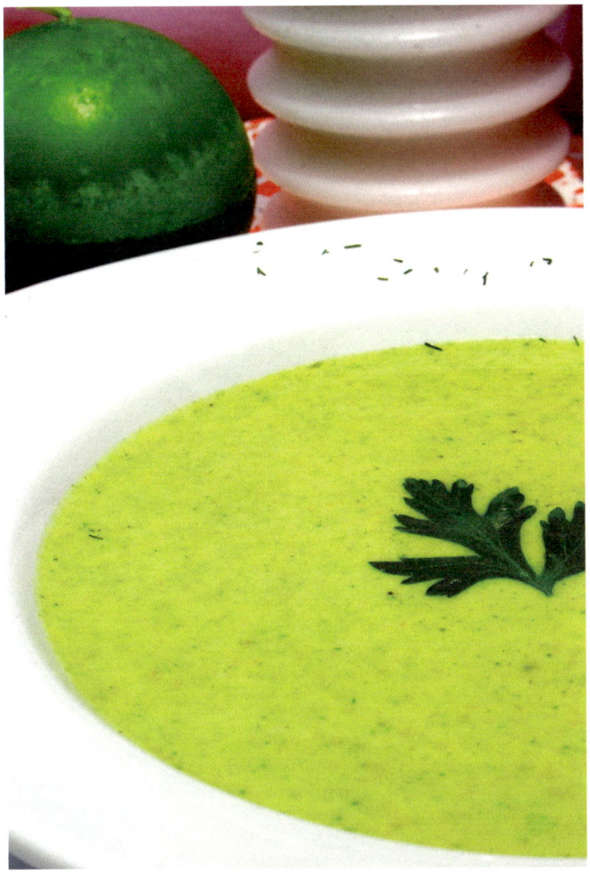

Serves 2
Preparation time: 20 minutes
Degree of difficulty: 2

3	CREAM OF MIXED VEGETABLE SOUP			
	Ingredients for 2 portions	**Equivalences**		**Calories**
■	½ cup chopped carrots			15.00
■	½ cup broccoli, cut into pieces			13.95
■	½ cup peas			37.00
■	½ cup skim milk			50.00
■	¼ cup water (optional)			0.00
■	1 sprig parsley, for garnishing			0.00
■	a pinch of salt and pepper			0.40
		Total Calories		**116.35**

→ Blanch vegetables. → Purée all ingredients in a blender (add water only if necessary). Place in a medium sized pan and heat over low. → Stir constantly until it thickens. → Season with salt and pepper. → Remove pan from heat and add warm milk. → Add salt to taste and garnish with parsley. → Serve warm.

see blanching vegetables

4. TOMATO AND THYME SOUP

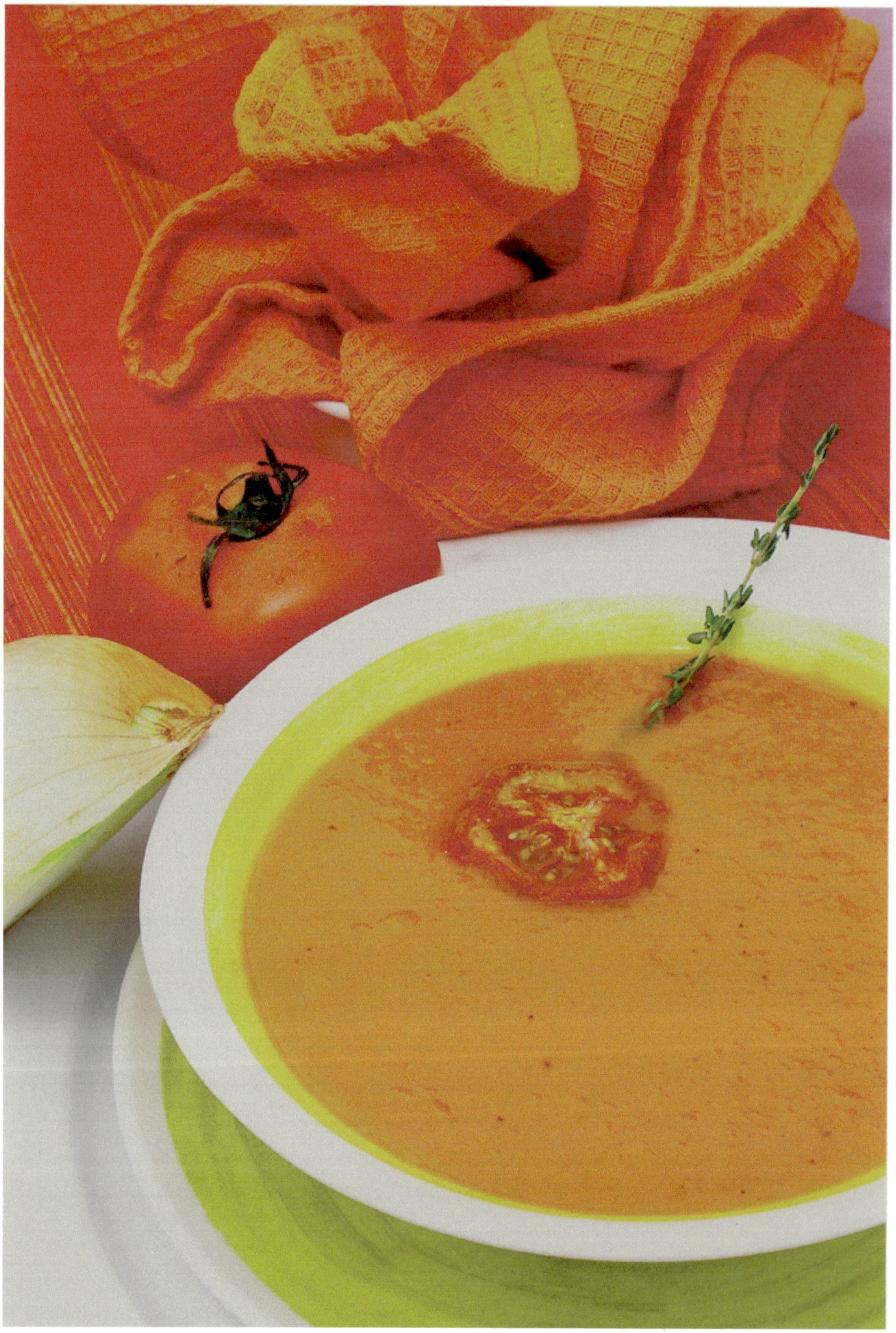

Serves 2
Preparation time: 10 minutes
Degree of difficulty: 2

4	TOMATO AND THYME SOUP			
	Ingredients for 2 portions	**Equivalences**		**Calories**
▪	4 ripe medium sized tomatoes, peeled, seeded, cut into pieces	2	cups	27.50
▪	2 sprigs fresh thyme or ½ teaspoon powdered thyme			0.00
▪	¼ cup carrots, chopped			19.00
▪	¼ celery stalk, diced			3.47
▪	¼ cup white onion, shredded			4.70
▪	1 ¼ cups boiling water			0.00
▪	1 teaspoon splenda or			0.00
	2 teaspoons brown sugar			40.00
▪	½ tablespoon extra-virgin olive oil			67.00
▪	1 slice dehydrated tomato, for garnishing			0.02
▪	a pinch of salt and pepper			0.40
		Total Calories		**162.09**

→ Heat oil in a pot over medium heat and add shredded onion. → Sauté onion until golden. → Add tomatoes. → Wait until tomatoes dissolve. → Add boiling water, carrots, celery and thyme sprigs and continue cooking for 2 minutes. → Season with salt and pepper. → Remove from heat and add splenda or brown sugar (to reduce the acidity of the tomato). → Discard thyme sprigs. → Blend and reheat in a pan for 1 more minute. → Remove from heat. → Salt to taste and garnish with dehydrated tomato. → Serve warm.

see peeling raw tomatoes
see sautéing

SANDWICHES

***Note:** The side of the bread that is spread with mayonnaise, mustard or butter is to be in contact with the ingredients of the sandwiches.*

1. CAPRESE SANDWICH

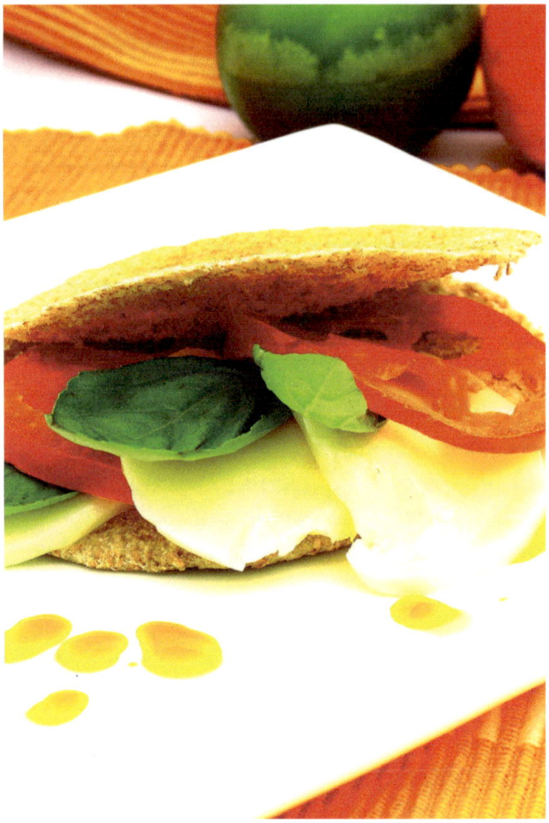

Serves 1
Preparation time: 5 minutes
Degree of difficulty: 1

1	**CAPRESE SANDWICH**			
	Ingredients for 1 portion	**Equivalences**		**Calories**
▪	1 whole wheat pita bread, cut in half			22.80
▪	2 or 3 thin slices low fat mozzarella cheese	¼	cup	22.50
▪	2 tomato slices, seeded			0.30
▪	3 fresh basil leaves			0.00
▪	1 teaspoon extra virgin olive or avocado oil			45.00
▪	a pinch of salt and pepper			0.40
		Total Calories		**91.00**

→ Put mozzarella cheese, tomato and basil in a bowl and season with extra virgin olive oil. → Add salt and pepper. → Fill pita bread with preparation. → Serve immediately.

2. OLIVE AND HARD-BOILED EGG SANDWICH

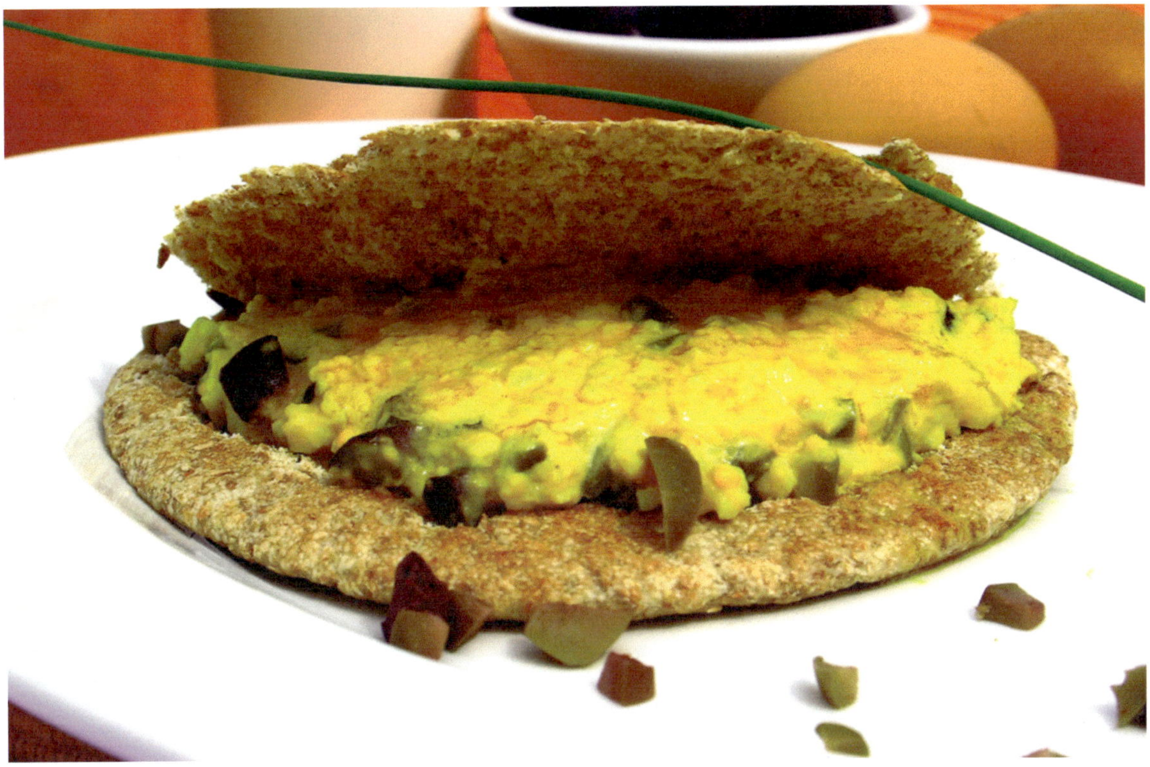

Serves 1
Preparation time: 7 minutes
Degree of difficulty: 1

2	OLIVE AND HARD-BOILED EGG SANDWICH			
	Ingredients for 1 portion	**Equivalences**		**Calories**
▪	1 whole wheat pita bread, cut in half			22.80
▪	6 green or black olives, pitted, finely chopped			108.00
▪	1 hard boiled egg, peeled, preferably *Omega-3* egg			90.00
▪	1 teaspoon Dijon mustard			0.00
▪	1 tablespoon *Homemade Mayonnaise*			127.35
▪	¼ teaspoon onion powder			0.00
▪	a pinch of salt and pepper			0.40
		Total Calories		**348.55**

→ Mash hard boiled egg and chopped olives with a fork. → Mix mayonnaise with powdered onion and mustard. → Mix all making it creamy. → Season with salt and pepper to taste. → Fill pita bread with preparation. → Serve immediately.

see Homemade Mayonnaise

3. TUNA SANDWICH

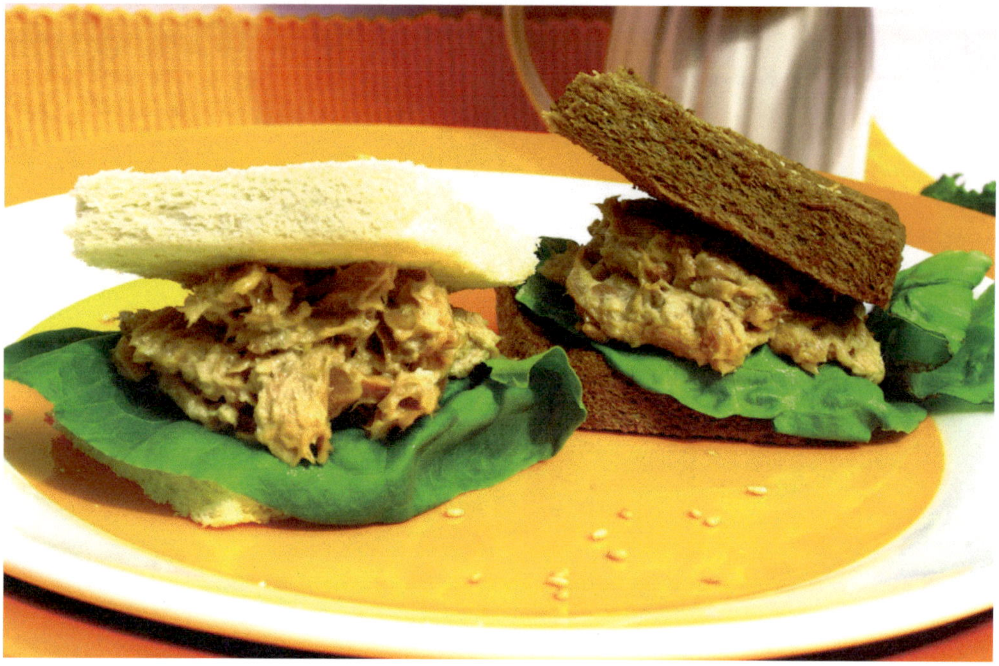

Serves 1
Preparation time: 5 minutes
Degree of difficulty: 1

3	TUNA SANDWICH			
	Ingredients for 1 portion	**Equivalences**		**Calories**
▪	2 slices low calorie whole wheat or white bread			90.00
▪	½ can tuna, packed in water and drained			140.00
▪	1 leaf lettuce, washed and pulled gently dry			1.60
▪	1 tablespoon *Homemade Mayonnaise*			127.35
▪	1 tablespoon mustard			0.00
▪	a pinch of salt and pepper			0.40
		Total Calories		**359.35**

→ Drain the tuna and mix in a bowl with the *Homemade Mayonnaise*. → Add salt to taste. → Spread mustard on one side of bread slices. → Place lettuce on the side spread with mustard and add tuna. → Place the other slice of bread on top. → May be prepared in advance on the same day it will be eaten. → Wrap and refrigerate until ready to eat.

see Homemade Mayonnaise

Note: makes a great packed lunch

4. EGG AND CHIVE SANDWICH

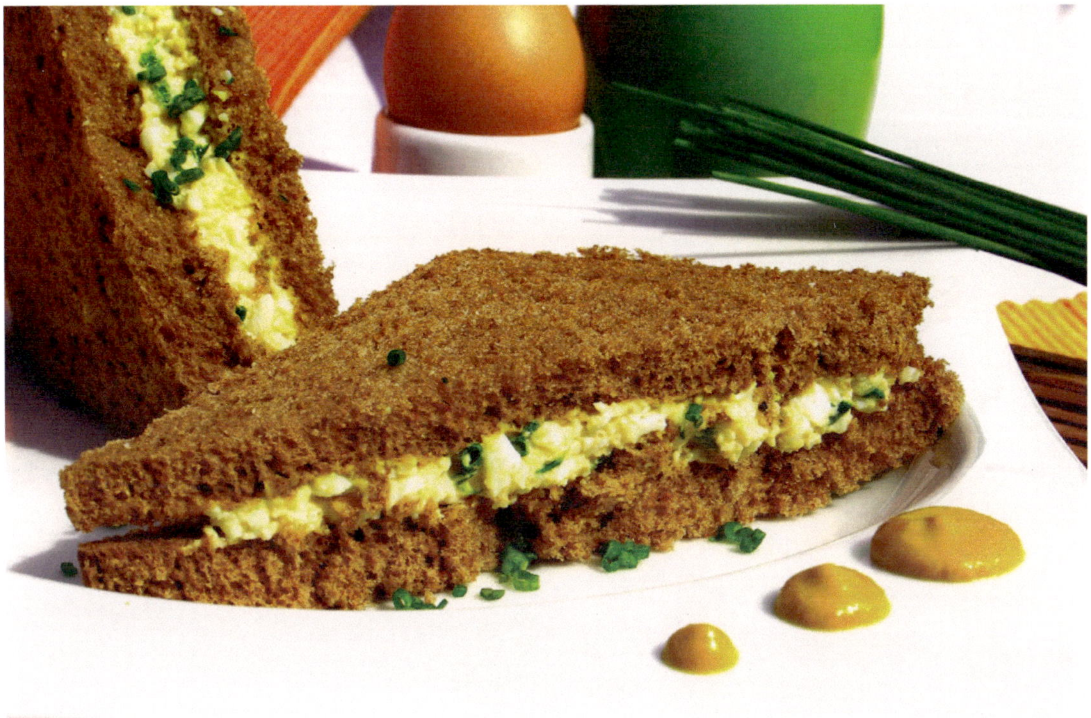

Serves 1
Preparation time: 7 minutes
Degree of difficulty: 1

4	EGG AND CHIVE SANDWICH			
	Ingredients for 1 portion	**Equivalences**		**Calories**
▪	2 slices low calorie whole wheat bread			90.00
▪	1 hard boiled egg, peeled, preferably *Omega-3* egg			90.00
▪	3 chives stalks, finely chopped			0.00
▪	1 teaspoon *Homemade Mayonnaise*			127.35
▪	1 teaspoon Dijon mustard			0.00
▪	a pinch of salt and pepper, to taste			0.40
		Total Calories		**307.75**

→ Peel the egg, place in a bowl and mash with a fork. → Add *Homemade Mayonnaise* and chopped chives. → Mix well and season with salt and pepper. → Spread mustard on one side bread.→ Add egg preparation on that side. → Place the other slice of bread on top. → May be prepared in advance on the same day it will be eaten. → Wrap and refrigerate until ready to eat.

see Homemade Mayonnaise

5. TURKEY OR HAM SANDWICH

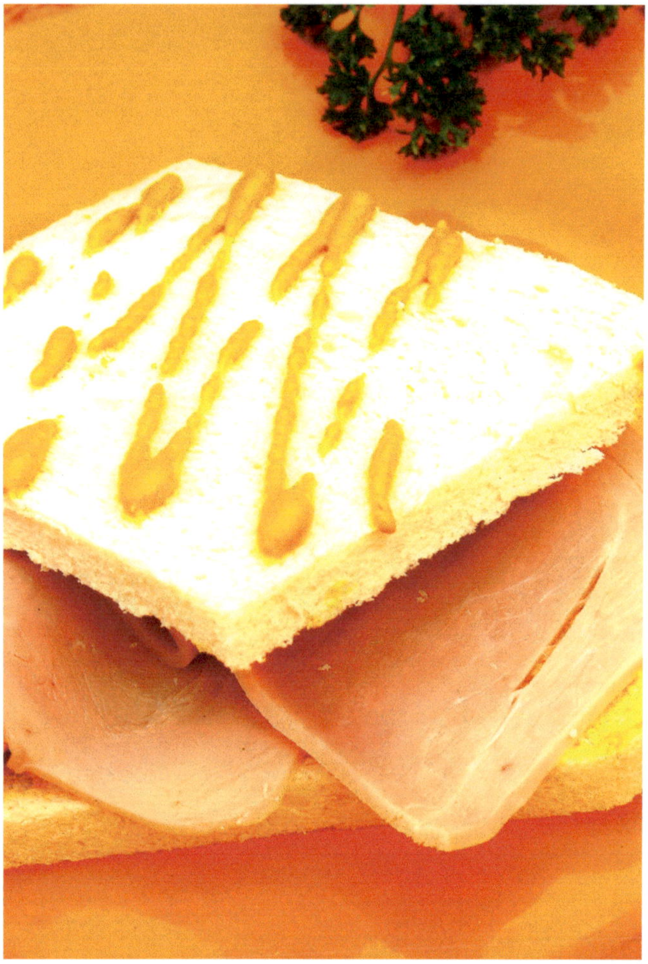

Serves 1
Preparation time: 3 minutes
Degree of difficulty: 1

5	TURKEY OR HAM SANDWICH			
	Ingredients for 1 portion	**Equivalences**		**Calories**
▪	2 slices low-calorie whole wheat bread			90.00
▪	1 slice turkey or lean ham deli meat	20 g	0.70 oz	19.20
▪	1 teaspoon Dijon mustard			0.00
		Total Calories		**109.20**

→ Spread Dijon mustard on one slice.→ Place turkey or ham on that side. → Place the other slice of bread on top. → May be prepared in advance on the same day it will be eaten. → Wrap and refrigerate until ready to eat.

6. CHICKEN SANDWICH

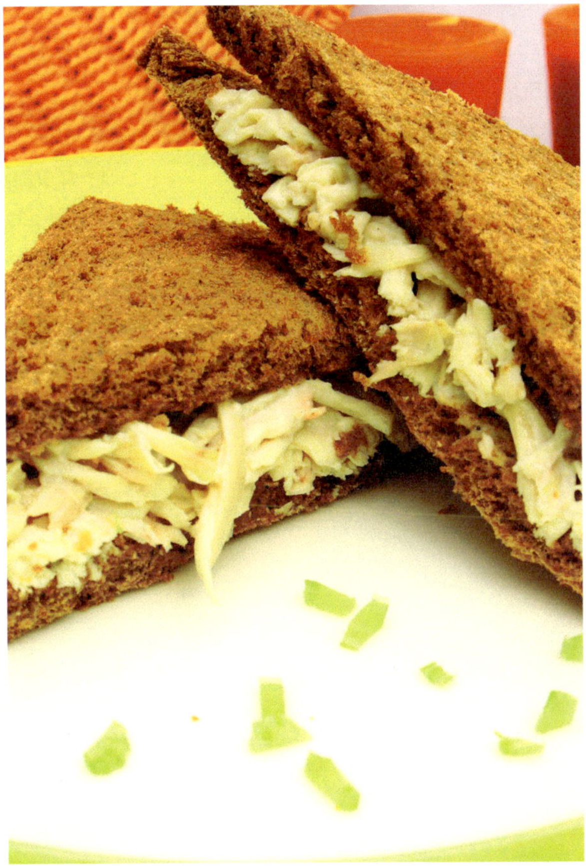

Serves 1
Preparation time: 10 minutes
Chicken breast cooking time: 20 minutes
Degree of difficulty: 2

6	CHICKEN SANDWICH			
	Ingredients for 1 portion	**Equivalences**		**Calories**
■	2 slices low-calorie white or whole wheat bread			90.00
■	¼ chicken breast, parboiled and pulled apart	90 g	3.15 oz	121.20
■	1 tablespoon *Homemade Mayonnaise*			127.35
■	1 teaspoon finely chopped celery			0.70
■	a pinch of salt and pepper			0.40
		Total Calories		**339.65**

→ In a bowl mix together the shredded chicken, finely chopped celery and *Homemade Mayonnaise*. → Season with salt and pepper to taste. → Spread mustard on one side of bread slices. → Cover chicken preparation on the side spread with mustard. → Cover other slice of bread on top. → May be prepared in advance on the same day it will be eaten. → Wrap and refrigerate until ready to eat.

see Chicken Breast Broth
see Homemade Mayonnaise

7. SALMON SANDWICH

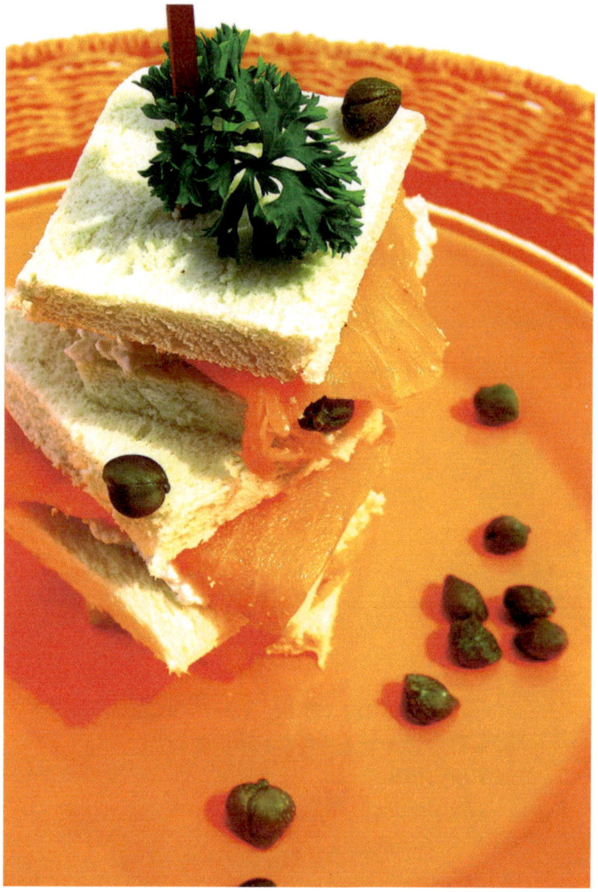

Serves 1
Preparation time: 7 minutes
Degree of difficulty: 1

7	SALMON SANDWICH			
	Ingredients for 1 portion	Equivalences		Calories
▪	2 slices low-calorie white or whole wheat bread			90.00
▪	2 slices smoked salmon (¼ cup)	40 g	1.4 oz	185.00
▪	2 teaspoons low fat ricotta or low fat cream cheese			8.33
▪	5 capers			0.00
▪	1 teaspoon extra-virgin olive or avocado oil *			134.00
▪	½ tablespoon lemon juice, to taste			0.80
▪	a pinch of salt and pepper			0.00
*	or any other gourmet oil of your choice	Total Calories		**418.13**

→ Place salmon slices in a bowl and add lemon juice, oil and capers. → Marinate for 2 minutes. → Season with salt and pepper to taste. → Spread cheese on one side of bread slices. → Place salmon and capers on the side spread with cheese. → Place with the other slice of bread on top. → Serve immediately.

8. TOMATO AND AVOCADO SANDWICH

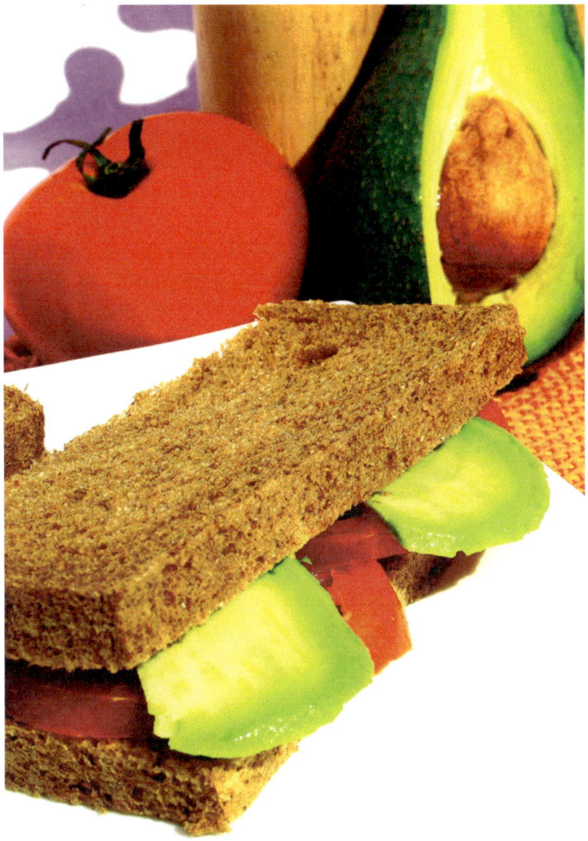

Serves 1
Preparation time: 7 minutes
Degree of difficulty: 1

8	TOMATO AND AVOCADO SANDWICH			
	Ingredients for 1 portion	**Equivalences**		**Calories**
▪	2 slices low-calorie whole wheat bread			90.00
▪	3 thin slices tomato, peeled and seeded	¼	cup	6.80
▪	¼ avocado, cut into slices			142.00
▪	¼ tablespoon lemon juice, to taste			0.40
▪	1 tablespoon *Homemade Mayonnaise*			127.35
▪	a pinch of salt and pepper			0.40
		Total Calories		**366.95**

→ Place the freshly cut avocado in a bowl and add lemon juice. → Season with salt and pepper to taste. → Set aside. → Spread *Homemade Mayonnaise* on one slice of bread. → Place tomato and avocado slices on that side. → Place the other slice of bread on top. → Serve immediately.

see Homemade Mayonnaise

9. HAM AND CHEESE SANDWICH

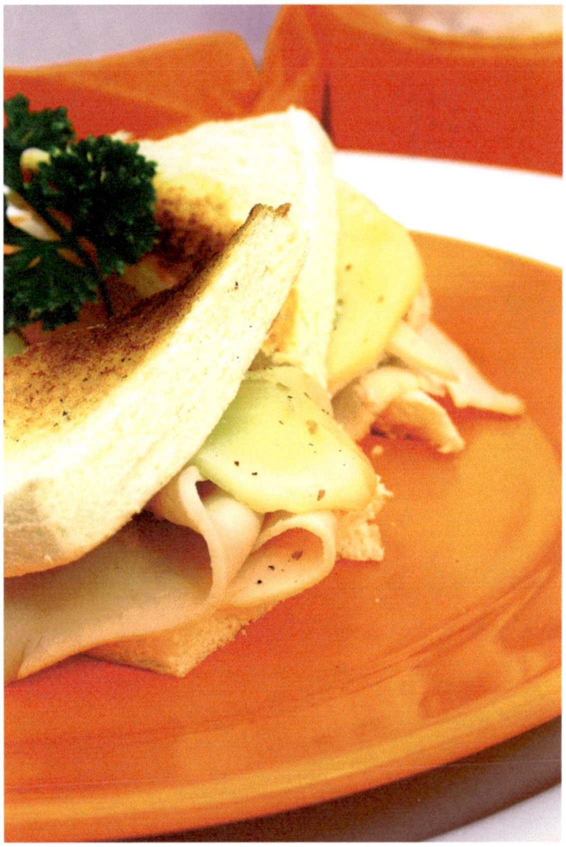

Serves 1
Preparation time: 5 minutes
Degree of difficulty: 1

9	HAM AND CHEESE SANDWICH			
	Ingredients for 1 portion	**Equivalences**		**Calories**
▪	2 slices low-calorie white or whole wheat bread			90.00
▪	1 slice low-fat fresh mozzarella cheese			45.00
▪	1 slice ham, trimmed of fat	20 g	0.70 oz	19.20
▪	1 teaspoon butter			37.00
		Total Calories		**191.20**

Preheat oven: 390º F – 200º C

→ Butter one side of bread slices. → Place cheese and ham on the side spread with butter. → Cover with the other slice. → Bake on a rack in the in oven for 2 ½ minutes or until bread is slightly golden. → Serve warm and eat immediately.

Culinary note: can also be eaten cold without using the oven.

MAIN COURSES

1. EGGPLANT A LA BOLOGNESE

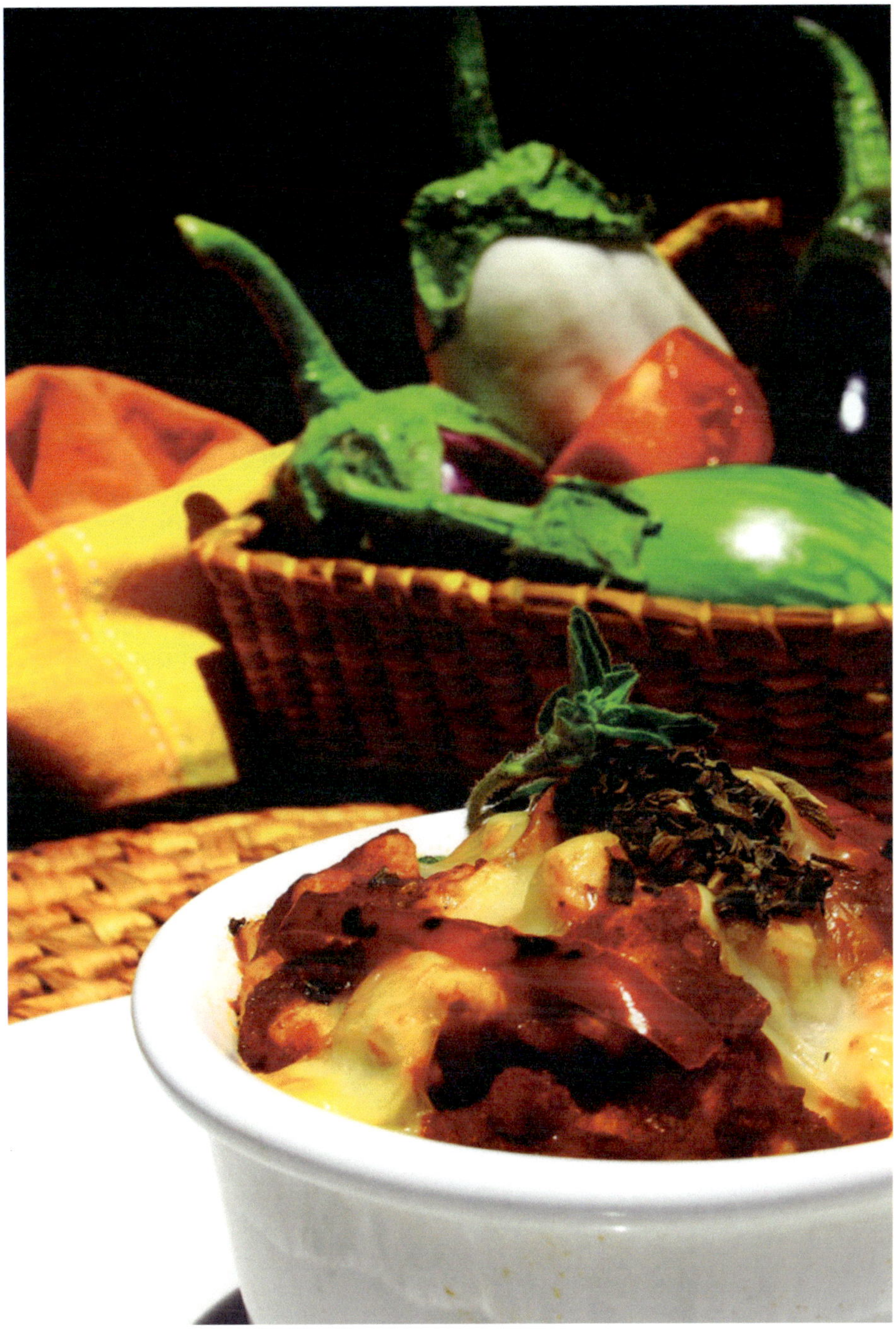

Serves 2
Preparation time: 20 minutes
Degree of difficulty: 2

1	EGGPLANT A LA BOLOGNESE (ITALIAN)			
	Ingredients for 2 portions	**Equivalences**		**Calories**
■	1 cup fat free ground chicken	125 g	4.3 oz	336.70
■	2 medium-sized eggplants approx.	2	cups	33.12
■	½ cup *Basic Tomato Sauce* without chicken			152.00
■	1 peeled red pepper cut into long strips* approx.	1	cup	20.80
■	4 thin slices of low fat mozzarella cheese approx.	½	cup	90.00
■	½ tablespoon dried whole oregano			0.00
■	1 tablespoon extra virgin olive oil			134.00
■	a pinch of salt and pepper			0.40
*	set aside 3 strips of red pepper for garnish	**Total Calories**		**767.02**

Preheat oven to 390º F-200º C.

→ Slice eggplant in circles, ¼ inch thickness and wash. → Heat oil in a non-stick frying pan. → Brown eggplants and peppers. → Remove from pan and set aside. → In the same pan, sauté ground chicken and mix with *Basic Tomato Sauce*. → Season with salt and pepper and set aside. → Make a layer of eggplant in a small baking dish. → Add a layer of peppers and pour one have of the tomato sauce with chicken on top. → Repeat alternating layers, as explained above. → Cover with 2 slices of mozzarella cheese and oregano. → Garnish with thin red pepper strips. → Bake for 10 minutes or until bubbly. → Serve warm.

see Basic Tomato Sauce
see washing eggplants
see browning
see sautéing
see gratinéing

2. CHICKEN OR TURKEY BURGER

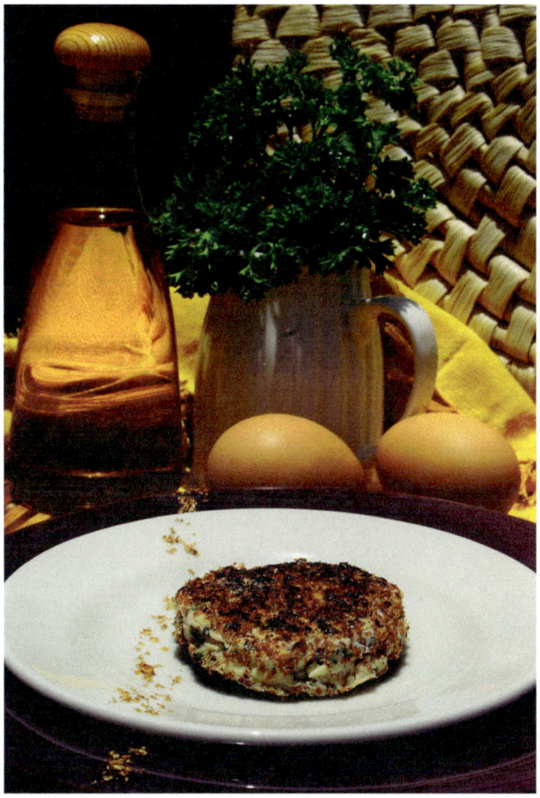

Serves 2
Preparation time: 10 minutes
Degree of difficulty: 1

2	CHICKEN OR TURKEY BURGER			
	Ingredients for 2 portions	**Equivalences**		**Calories**
▪	½ cup ground chicken or turkey , fat free (no skin or fat)	125 g	4.3 oz	168.35
▪	1 teaspoon chopped parsley			0.00
▪	1 egg white, preferably *Omega-3* egg			10.60
▪	½ tablespoon extra-virgin olive or avocado oil			67.00
▪	¼ cup whole wheat bread crumbs			45.00
▪	a pinch of salt and pepper			0.40
		Total Calories		**291.35**

→ Season ground chicken or turkey with salt, pepper and parsley mix well. → Form patties and set aside. → Beat egg white lightly in a bowl using a fork. → Place bread crumbs in a flat dish. → Dip both sides of burgers in the beaten egg white. → Turn burgers in bread crumbs until coated. → Heat oil in a non-stick frying pan and fry burgers. → Remove burgers from heat when brown and cooked. → Allow to rest briefly on paper towel to absorb excess fat. → Serve warm. → If you wish, serve the burger with a salad or ½ cup of *Country-Style Mashed Potatoes.*

see frying

3. BREADED CHICKEN OR TURKEY CUTLETS (MILANESE)

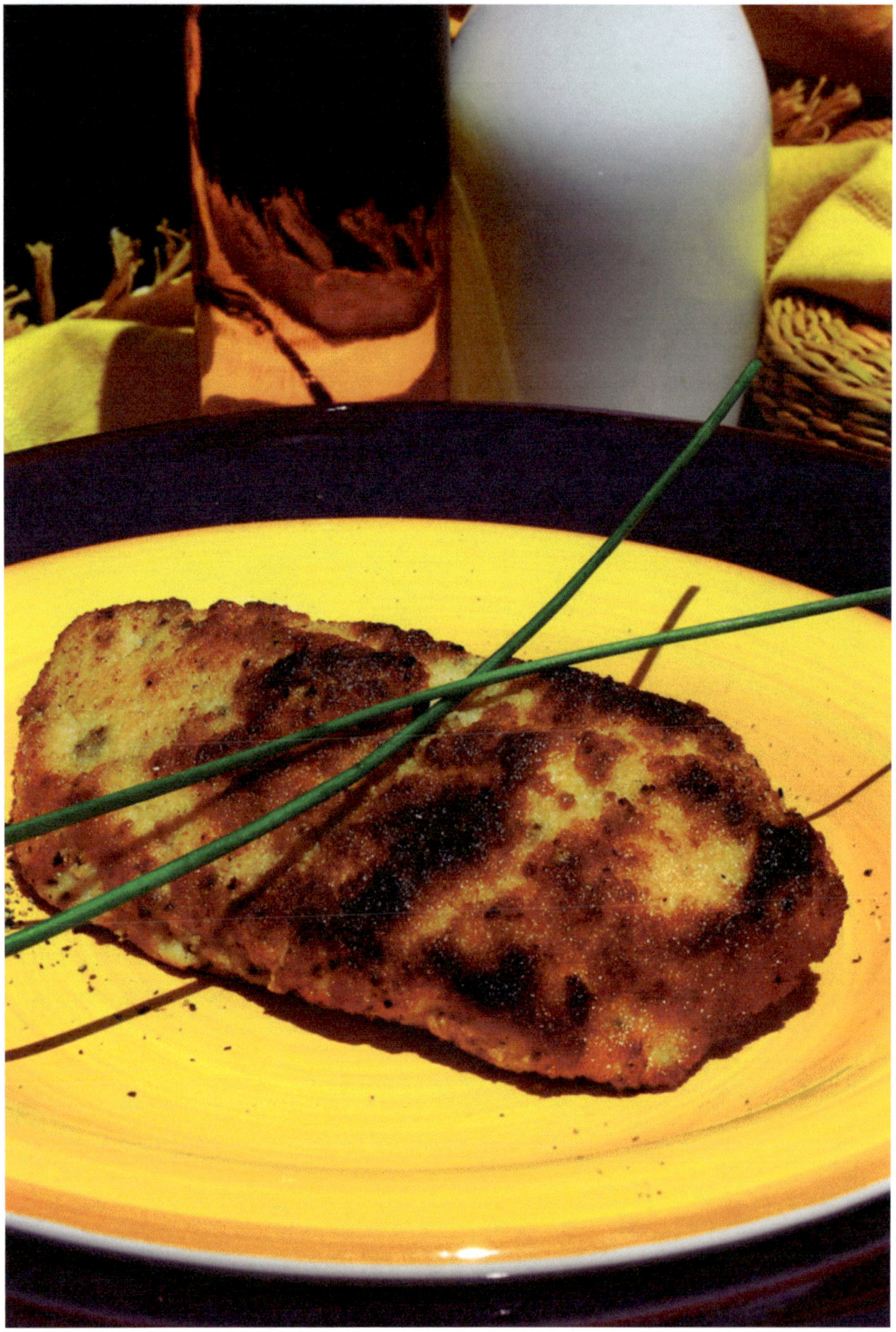

Serves 2
Preparation time: 10 minutes
Degree of difficulty: 1

3	BREADED CHICKEN OR TURKEY CUTLETS			
	Ingredients for 2 portions	**Equivalences**		**Calories**
■	2 medium-sized skinless chicken breast filets or	120 g	4.2 oz	242.00
	2 medium-sized turkey filets	120 g	4.2 oz	168.35
■	2 whole wheat crackers, ground			40.00
■	1 egg white, preferably *Omega-3* egg			10.60
■	½ tablespoon extra-virgin olive or avocado oil			67.00
■	a pinch of salt and pepper			0.40
		Total Calories		**528.35**

→ Season filets with salt and pepper. → Beat egg white lightly in a bowl using a fork. → Place ground crackers in a flat dish. → Dip both sides of filets in the beaten egg white. → Turn filets in ground crackers until coated. → Heat oil in a non-stick frying pan and fry filets. → Remove from heat when brown and cooked. → Allow to rest on paper towel to absorb excess fat. → Serve warm. → If you wish, serve the cutlets with *Hot Vegetables* or ½ cup of *Spinach Purée* per person.

see frying

4. CURRY CHICKEN WITH MINT

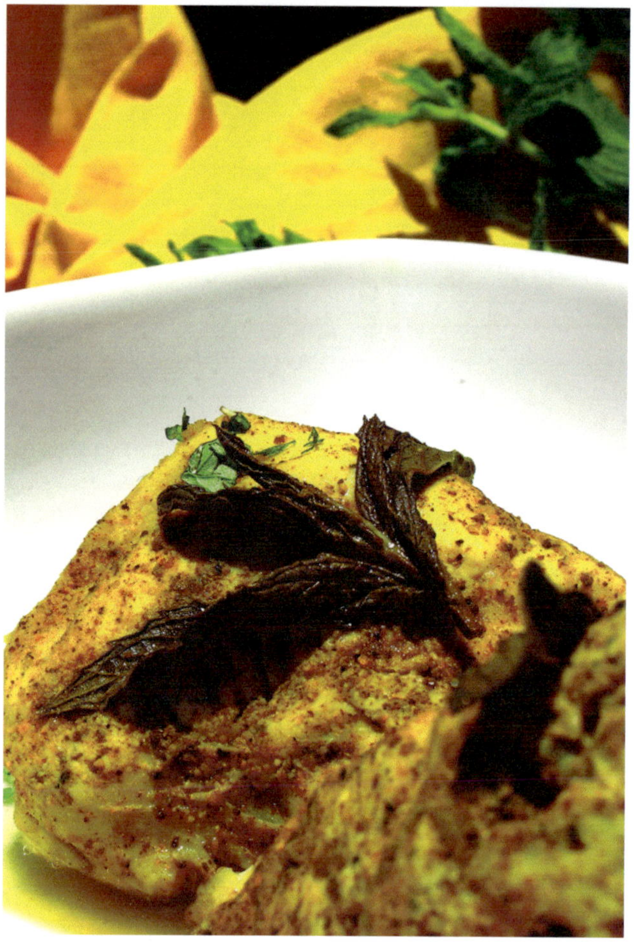

Serves 2
Preparation time: 35 minutes
Degree of difficulty: 1

4	CURRIED CHICKEN WITH MINT			
	Ingredients for 2 portions	**Equivalences**		**Calories**
▪	1 medium-sized chicken breast, boneless and skinless (1½ cup)	360 g	12.6 oz	484.00
▪	½ teaspoon curry			0.00
▪	1 sprig of fresh mint			0.00
▪	a pinch of salt and pepper			0.40
		Total Calories		**484.40**

Preheat oven to 350° F - 180° C.

→ Split chicken breast into halves. → Season with salt and pepper and sprinkle with curry. → Place the 2 halves in a baking pan. → Place whole mint leaves on top and cover pan with aluminum foil. → Bake for approximately 30 minutes or until chicken is done. → Serve warm with a salad or ½ baked potato per person.

5. BAKED CHICKEN WITH ROSEMARY

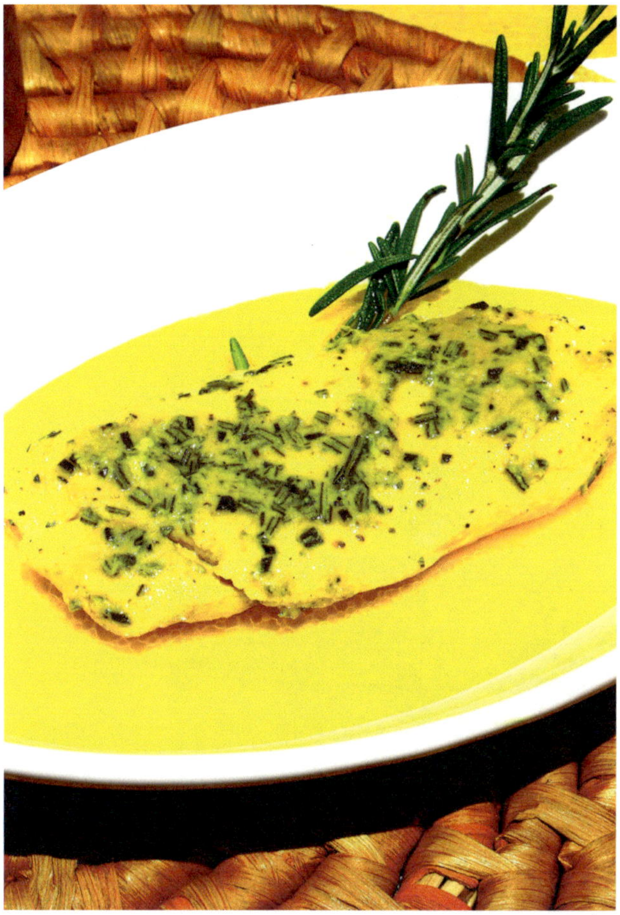

Serves 2
Preparation time: 35 minutes
Degree of difficulty: 1

5	BAKED CHICKEN WITH ROSEMARY			
	Ingredients for 2 portions	**Equivalences**		**Calories**
▪	1 medium sized chicken breast, boneless and skinless (1½ cup)	360 g	12.6 oz	484.00
▪	1 tablespoon mustard			0.00
▪	1 teaspoon rosemary			0.00
▪	a pinch of salt and pepper			0.40
		Total Calories		**484.40**

Preheat oven to 350º F - 180º C.

→ Split the chicken breast in two and season both sides with mustard, rosemary, salt and pepper.→ Place in a baking dish. → Cover dish with aluminum foil. →Bake for approximately 30 minutes or until chicken is done. → Serve warm with vegetables or ½ cup of brown rice with vegetables per person.

6. NEAPOLITAN-STYLE BAKED CHICKEN

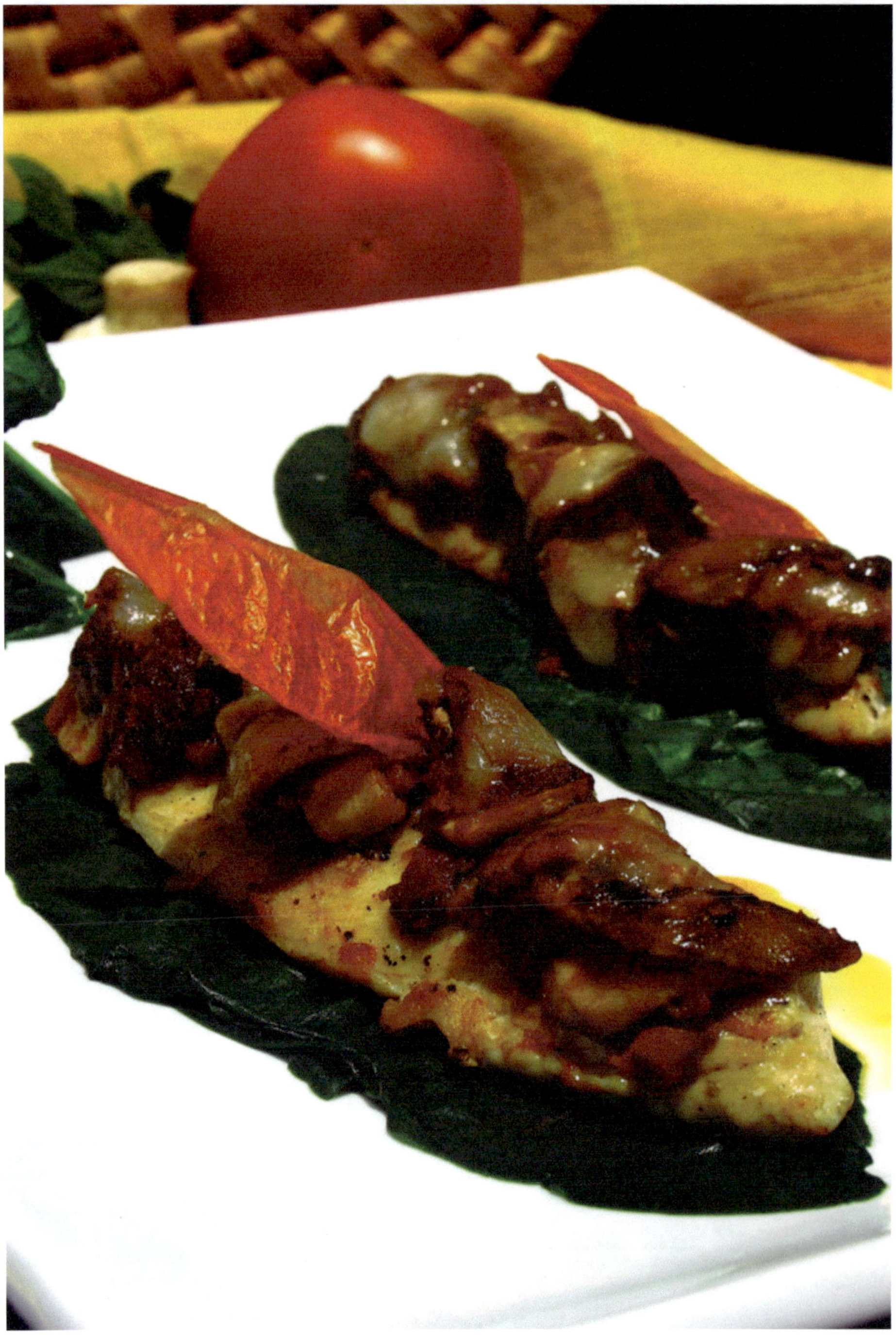

Serves 2
Preparation time: 25 minutes
Degree of difficulty: 2

6	NAPOLITAN-STYLE BAKED CHICKEN			
	Ingredients for 2 portions	**Equivalences**		**Calories**
▪	1 medium-sized chicken breast, boneless and skinless (1½ cup)	360 g	12.6 oz	484.00
▪	1 cup chopped spinach			4.40
▪	½ cup sliced mushrooms			20.00
▪	3 tablespoons *Basic Tomato Sauce* without chicken			5.80
▪	1 teaspoon minced garlic (optional)			
▪	1 tablespoon extra virgin olive or avocado oil			134.00
▪	¼ cup low fat mozzarella cheese, shredded			45.00
▪	1 teaspoon dried oregano			0.00
▪	a pinch of salt and pepper			0.40
		Total Calories		**693.60**

Preheat oven to 350° F - 180° C.

→ Cut chicken breast into 4 equal-size filets. → Heat oil in a non-stick frying pan. → Brown both sides of chicken filets. → Remove from pan when half cooked and set aside. → In the same frying pan, sauté garlic and sliced mushrooms. → Add *Basic Tomato Sauce* and season with salt and pepper. → Set aside. → Blanch spinach and drain well. → Place spinach in a baking dish and top with chicken filets. → Cover filets with the reserved preparation of tomato sauce, mushroom and garlic. → Top with shredded mozzarella cheese and oregano. → Bake for approximately 15 minutes or until chicken is completely cooked and cheese is bubbly. → Serve warm.

see Basic Tomato Sauce
see browning
see sautéing
see blanching vegetables
see gratinéing

7. CHICKEN SAUTÉ WITH VEGETABLES

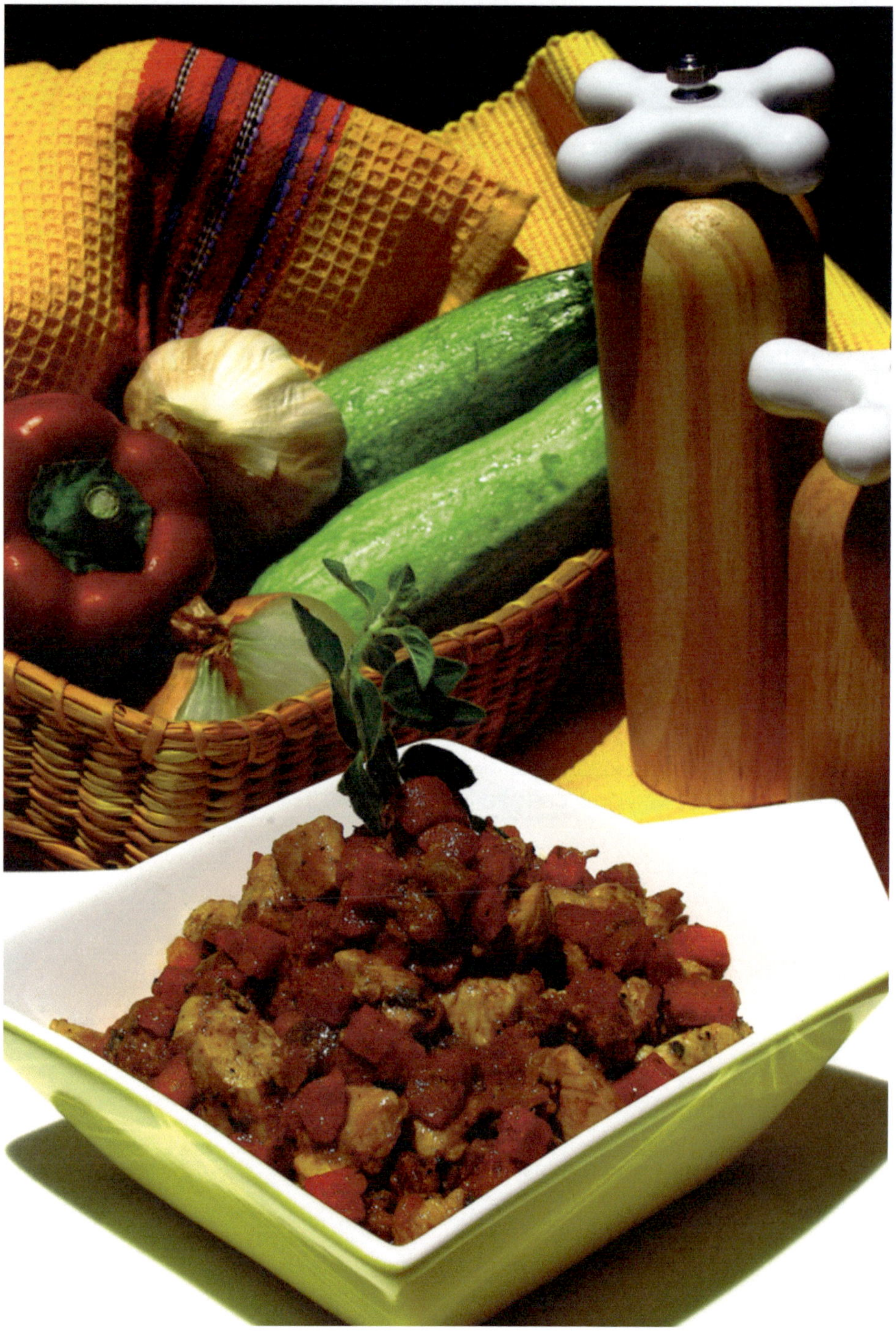

Serves 2
Preparation time: 25 minutes
Degree of difficulty: 2

7	CHICKEN SAUTÉ WITH VEGETABLES			
	Ingredients for 2 portions	**Equivalences**		**Calories**
■	1 medium-sized chicken breast, boneless and skinless (1½ cup)	360 g	12.6 oz	484.00
■	1 cup white onion, diced			16.30
■	½ cup tomatoes peeled, seeded and diced			13.70
■	1 cup zucchini seeded and diced			29.50
■	½ cup red pepper peeled, seeded and diced	½	cup	10.40
■	½ teaspoon dried oregano			0.00
■	a pinch of cumin			0.00
■	1 teaspoon low sodium soy sauce			10.00
■	1 tablespoon apple cider vinegar			0.60
■	½ teaspoon minced garlic			2.50
■	1 tablespoon extra virgin olive or avocado oil			134.00
■	a pinch of salt and pepper			0.40
		Total Calories		**701.40**

→ Prepare in a bowl a sauce with soy, vinegar, oregano, cumin, salt and pepper. → Marinate chicken in the sauce for 10 minutes. → Set aside. → Heat oil in a non-stick frying pan. → Lightly brown the garlic and onion. → Remove from pan and set aside. → Place marinated chicken in the hot frying pan and sear on both sides. → Reduce heat to low. → Add browned onion and garlic. → Add tomato, zucchini, pepper, and sauté. → Add marinade sauce to chicken. → Taste to verify appropriate saltiness. → Stir gently until liquid evaporates, vegetables are tender and chicken is done. → Serve warm.

see peeling raw tomatoes
see browning
see sautéing

8. GRILLED FISH IN PAPILLOTE

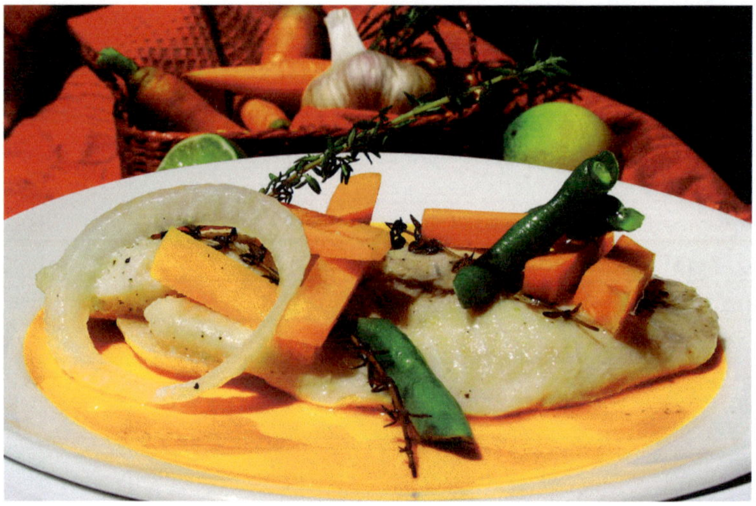

Serves 2
Preparation time: 30 minutes
Degree of difficulty: 3

8	GRILLED OR BAKED FISH IN PAPILLOTE			
	Ingredients for 2 portions	Equivalences		Calories
▪	2 white fish filets, boneless (sole, sea bass, grouper, shark, tilapia, etc.)	120 g	4.2 oz	97.40
▪	½ teaspoon chopped garlic			2.50
▪	½ tablespoon lemon juice, or the amount you wish			0.80
▪	2 tablespoons extra virgin olive or avocado oil*			268.00
▪	½ cup green beans, cut diagonally in half			14.30
▪	½ cup carrots, cut julienne style			19.00
▪	2 round slices of white onion			8.15
▪	2 sprigs fresh thyme			0.00
▪	a pinch of salt and pepper			0.40
▪	aluminum foil to wrap the fish as in an envelope (papillote).			
*	or any other gourmet oil of your choice	Total Calories		**410.55**

Preheat oven or grill to 390º F - 200º C.

→ Blanch and place carrots and green beans. → Season each filet with salt, pepper and garlic. → Separate the rings of the white onion and place on one end of aluminum foil. → Arrange fish on top of onion. → Squeeze lemon juice over filet. → Put thyme sprigs on top of filet. → Arrange blanched carrots and green beans on both sides. → Cover with the other end of the foil, and fold the edges together. → Wrap the other filet using the same technique. → Bake in oven or on grill for approximately 20 minutes or until fish is cooked. → Remove from heat and open envelope (papillote) carefully to allow steam to escape. → Serve warm.

see envelope (papillote)
see blanching vegetables

9. GRILLED FISH

Serves 2
Preparation time: 10 minutes (after marinating filets for 2 hours)
Degree of difficulty: 2

9	GRILLED FISH			
	Ingredients for 2 portions	**Equivalences**		**Calories**
▪	2 white fish filets (¼ pound)	120 g	4.2 oz	97.40
▪	2 tablespoons extra virgin olive or avocado oil			268.00
▪	2 garlic cloves, minced			10.00
▪	a pinch of salt and pepper			0.40
		Total Calories		**375.80**

Put oil and garlic in a bowl. → Mix well and season with salt and pepper. → Place fish filets in oil mix turf and marinate in the refrigerator for 1 hour. → Turn over filets and let stand for 1 more hour. → Put a griddle or non-stick frying pan over medium heat. → Place filets without oil. → Brown each side of filets for approximately 4 minutes or until fish is cooked. → Serve warm. → If desired, add a few drops of lemon and serve with a salad or rice.

see browning technique

10. MEDITERRANEAN SALMON

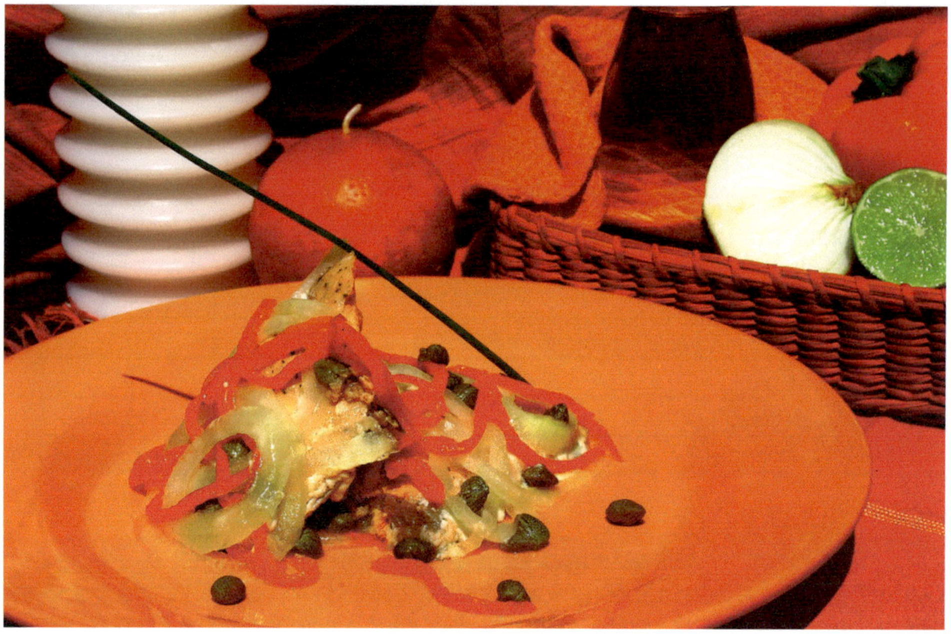

Serves 2
Preparation time: 25 minutes
Degree of difficulty: 2

10	MEDITERRANEAN SALMON			
	Ingredients for 2 portions	**Equivalences**		**Calories**
▪	2 medium-sized salmon filets	120 g	4.2 oz	215.70
▪	½ cup white onion, washed and thinly sliced			8.15
▪	1 red pepper peeled, seeded and cut into thin strips	1	cup	21.00
▪	10 capers	1	tbs.	1.45
▪	1 tablespoon extra virgin olive or avocado oil			134.00
▪	½ tablespoon lemon juice, adjust to taste	½	tbs.	0.80
▪	a pinch of pepper			0.00
▪	wrap aluminum foil			–
		Total Calories		**381.10**

Preheat oven to 350º F – 180º C

→ Season both sides of salmon filets with salt and pepper. → Place in one medium size or 2 individual baking pans. → Add peppers, onion and capers. → Sprinkle filets with olive oil. → Cover pans with aluminum foil. → Bake for approximately 20 minutes or until fish is fully cooked. → Serve warm with a few drops of lemon juice. → Serve with a salad or ½ baked potato per person.

11. EGGPLANT WITH OLIVES AU GRATIN (Bubbly)

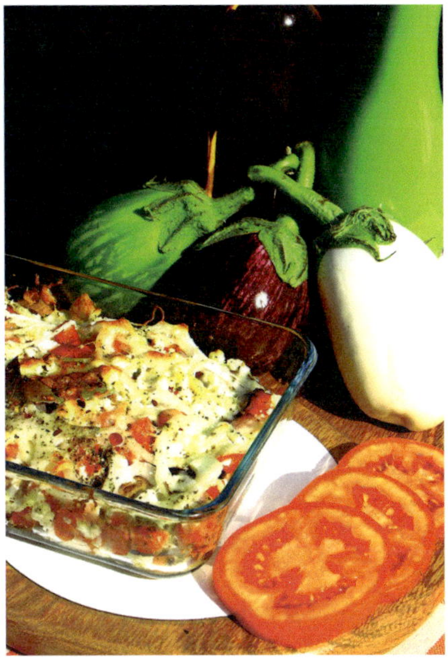

Serves 2
Preparation time: 25 minutes
Degree of difficulty: 3

11	**EGGPLANTS WITH OLIVES AU GRATEN**			
	Ingredients for 2 portions	**Equivalences**		**Calories**
■	2 medium sized eggplants, thinly sliced *	2	cups	33.12
■	1 medium sized white onion, washed and thinly sliced *	1	cup	16.30
■	½ cup tomatoes, peeled, seeded and diced			13.75
■	1 teaspoon minced garlic			5.60
■	1 dried bay leaf			0.00
■	10 black olives cut in halves	¼	cup	216.80
■	¼ cup low fat ricotta cheese, crumbled			50.00
■	1 teaspoon dried whole oregano			0.00
■	1 tablespoon extra virgin olive or avocado oil			134.00
■	a pinch of salt and pepper			0.40
*	cut into fine round slices	**Total Calories**		**469.97**

Preheat oven to 390º F – 200º C

→ Slice eggplants in circles and wash. → Place in a rectangular baking dish. → Cover with onion slices. → Place tomato, garlic, bay leaf, ricotta cheese and olives on top. → Spread ingredients evenly. → Season with salt and pepper. → Sprinkle with olive oil → Top with oregano. → Bake for 15 minutes or until cheese is bubbly. → Serve warm. → Serve with chicken or fish.

see peeling raw tomatoes
see washing eggplants
see gratinéing

12. PORK LOIN WITH SAGE

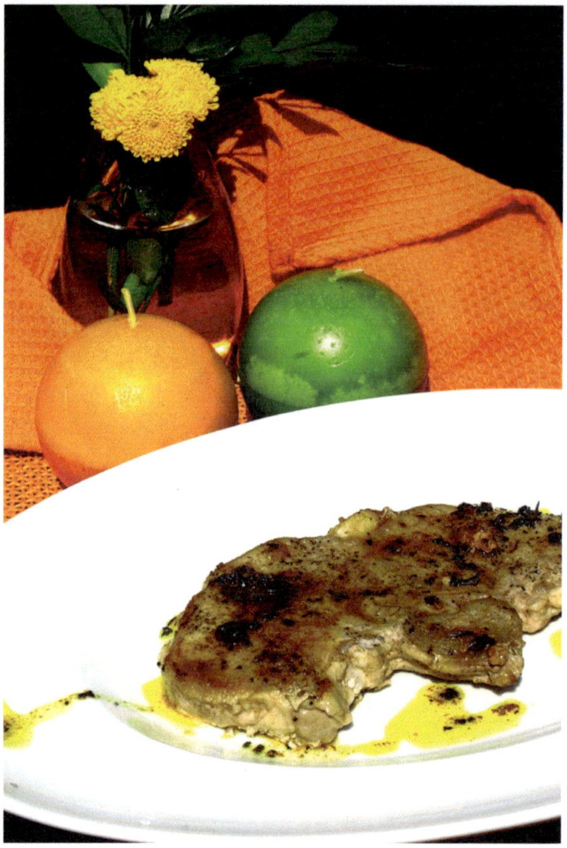

Serves 2
Preparation time: 10 minutes
Degree of difficulty: 2

12	PORK LOIN WITH SAGE			
	Ingredients for 2 portions	**Equivalences**		**Calories**
▪	2 lean pork loin filets or	120 g	4.2 oz	117.00
	2 lean pork chops	120 g	4.2 oz	246.00
▪	½ tablespoon extra-virgin olive or avocado oil			67.00
▪	½ tablespoon butter			55.55
▪	½ teaspoon dried sage			0.00
▪	a pinch of salt and pepper			0.40
		Total Calories		**485.95**

→ Season pork loins or chops with salt and pepper . → Heat oil in a non-stick frying pan. → Fry both sides of meat until well done. → Remove from heat and set aside. → Melt butter in frying pan over low heat. → Add sage and mix well. → Remove from heat before boiling. → Spread hot mix over meat. → Serve immediately. → Serve with salad or glazed carrots.

see frying

13. LENTILS WITH VEGETABLES

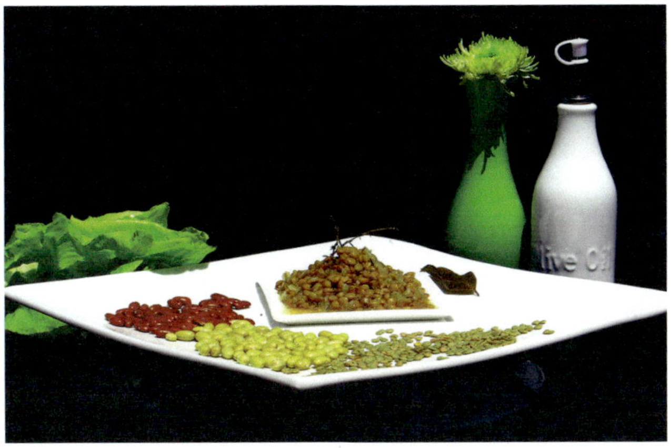

Serves 5
Preparation time: 40 minutes
Degree of difficulty: 3

13	LENTILS WITH VEGETABLES			
	Ingredients for 5 portions	**Equivalences**		**Calories**
▪	2 cups dry lentils sorted, washed and drained			1248.00
▪	½ cup white onion, washed and diced			8.15
▪	¼ cup carrots, diced			7.50
▪	¼ cup tomatoes, peeled, seeded and chopped			6.85
▪	1 tablespoon minced garlic			5.00
▪	1 small bay leaf			0.00
▪	1 tablespoon extra virgin olive or avocado oil*			134.00
▪	2 cups cold water, approximately			0.00
▪	a pinch of salt and pepper			0.40
*	or any other gourmet oil of your choice	**Total Calories**		**1409.90**

Cook lentils in advance, minimum cooking time 20 minutes. → Heat oil over medium heat in a medium-sized pot. → Add onion and brown. → Wait 1 minute, then add garlic and brown. → Add bay leaf, tomatoes and carrots. → Season with salt and pepper. → Sauté for 1 minute. → Add cooked lentils. → Mix gently and add salt to taste. → Serve warm, ½ cup of lentils per person, → Serve lentils with a salad of your choice.

To use cooked legumes another day, we suggest freezing it in individual portions when cool.

see peeling raw tomatoes
see washing and cooking legumes al dente
see browning
see sautéing

14. MACARONI WITH TOFU AND MUSHROOMS

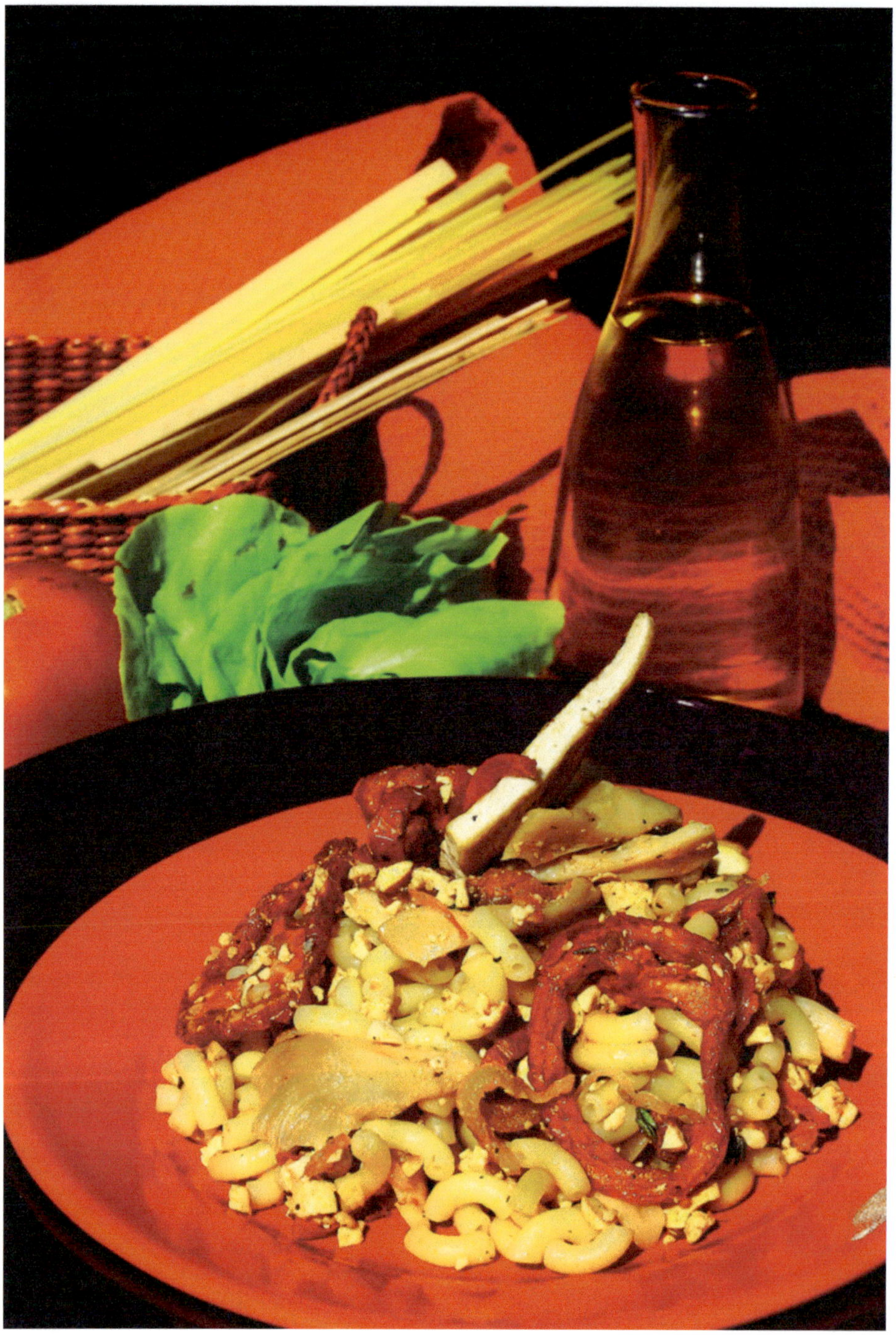

Serves 2
Preparation time: 20 minutes
Degree of difficulty: 3

14	MACARONI WITH TOFU AND MUSHROOMS			
	Ingredients for 2 portions	**Equivalences**		**Calories**
▪	½ cup uncooked macaroni			80.00
▪	½ cup tofu, cut into small cubes			39.00
▪	½ cup sliced mushrooms			8.98
▪	3 sundried tomatoes, cut into thin stripes			0.00
▪	1 garlic clove, minced			2.28
▪	½ cup white onion, in julienne slices			7.50
▪	1 medium sized tomato peeled and seeded and diced			18.10
▪	1 teaspoon dried oregano			0.00
▪	1 teaspoon thyme			0.00
▪	1 tablespoon extra virgin olive or avocado oil			134.00
▪	1 teaspoon butter			37.00
▪	a pinch of salt and pepper			0.40
		Total Calories		**327.26**

To prepare sauce:

→ Hydrate dried tomatoes. → Set aside. → Heat oil in a non-stick frying pan. → Slightly brown onion and garlic. → Add tofu and tomato. → Sauté for 1 minute. → Add thyme and stir. → Season with salt and pepper and add oregano. → Add mushrooms and hydrated tomatoes. → Mix gently and remove from heat. → Cover and keep warm in the frying pan.

To cook pasta:

→ Place a medium saucepan on the heat filled half full of with water. → Bring water a rolling boil and add ½ teaspoon of salt. → Add macaroni. → Cook for approximately 5 or 6 minutes or until pasta is *al dente*. → Remove from heat immediately and drain in a colander. → Arrange the pasta in a platter. → Add melted butter and mix the macaroni with a fork. → Add previously reserved hot sauce. → Mix gently with a fork. → Serve immediately, ¾ cup per person. → We suggest serving this dish with a light salad.

Note: You may substitute rice for macaroni or salad. Serve ½ sauce cup per person.

see hydrating sundried tomatoes
see peeling raw tomatoes
see browning
see sautéing
see cooking pasta al dente

15. SPAGHETTI WITH VEGETABLES AND OLIVES

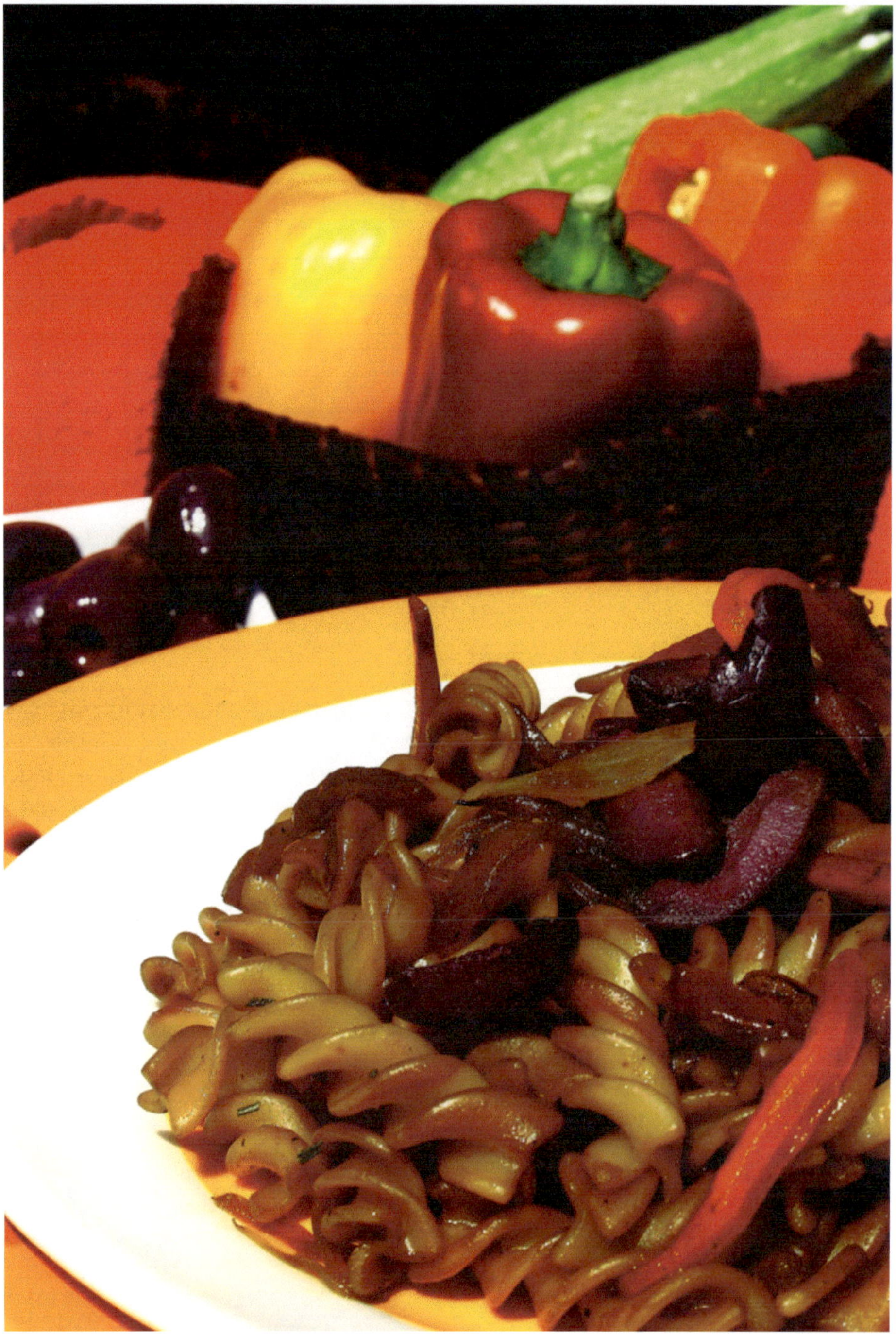

Serves 2
Preparation time: 20 minutes
Degree of difficulty: 3

15	SPAGHETTI WITH VEGETABLES AND OLIVES			
	Ingredients for 2 portions	Equivalences		Calories
▪	½ cup uncooked spaghetti			100.00
▪	1 cup zucchini, cut into thick strips			29.50
▪	1 cup carrots, cut into thick strips			30.00
▪	1 cup white onions, cut into thick strips			16.30
▪	1 cup lightly roasted red peppers, cut into thick strips			20.80
▪	10 black olives, cut into quarters	¼	cup	216.00
▪	4 tablespoons low sodium soy sauce			40.00
▪	1 tablespoon extra virgin olive or avocado oil			134.00
▪	a pinch of salt and pepper			0.40
		Total Calories		**587.00**

To prepare sauce:

→ Cut all vegetables to the same size. → Heat oil in a deep non-stick frying pan or wok. → Sauté carrots for 1 minute. → Add peppers and brown. → Add onion and zucchini. → Brown. → Add soy sauce and stir. → Cook al dente. → Add olives. → Season with salt and pepper. → Remove from heat. → Cover and set aside warm.

To cook pasta:

→ Place on fire a medium saucepan on heat and fill to the halfway mark. → Bring water to a rolling boil and add ½ teaspoon salt. → Add spaghetti. → Cook for 5 or 6 minutes or until pasta is *al dente*. → Remove from heat and drain. → Add spaghetti heated sauce. → Mix gently. → Arrange the pasta in a platter or on individual plates. → Serve warm, ¾ cup per person. → If you wish, serve pasta with a light salad.

see slightly roasting peppers
see sautéing
see browning
see cooking pasta al dente

16. ZUCCHINI AU GRATIN WITH MUSHROOMS

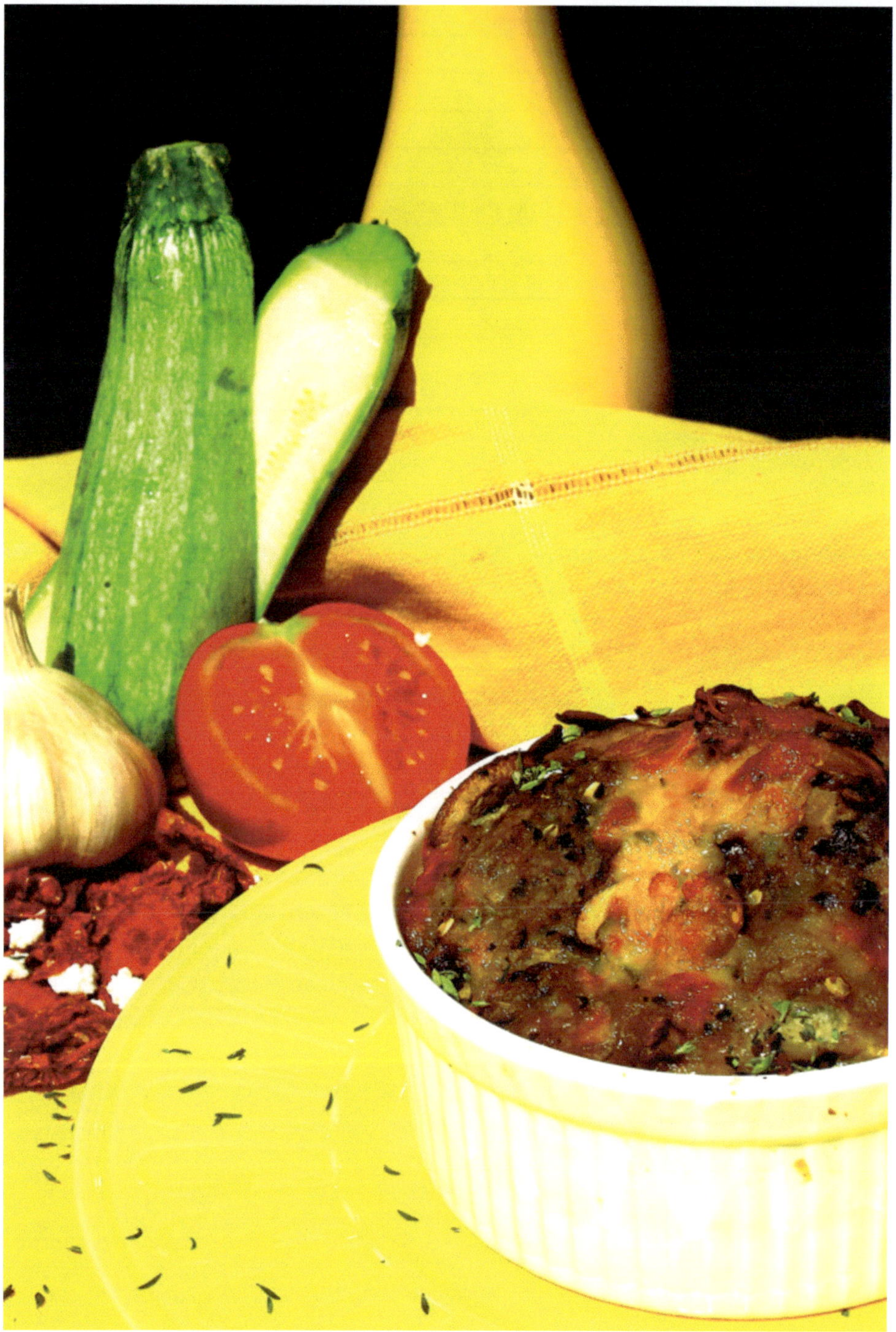

Serves 2
Preparation time: 30 minutes
Degree of difficulty: 2

16	ZUCCHINI AU GRATIN WITH MUSHROOMS			
	Ingredients for 2 portions	**Equivalences**		**Calories**
▪	2 cups zucchini, finely sliced, ¼ inch thick rounds			59.00
▪	½ cup mushrooms, sliced			8.98
▪	¼ cup low fat mozzarella cheese, shredded			22.50
▪	1 tablespoon tomato, peeled, seeded and chopped (optional)			5.50
▪	1 tablespoon whole garlic, minced			6.84
▪	½ teaspoon dried marjoram			0.00
▪	1 teaspoon chopped parsley			0.00
▪	1 tablespoon extra virgin olive or avocado oil			134.00
▪	a pinch of salt and pepper			0.40
		Total Calories		**237.22**

Preheat oven to 390º F – 200º C

→ Heat oil in a deep non stick frying pan or wok. → Add garlic and brown. → Add and sauté tomato, zucchini, parsley and marjoram. → Stir and season with salt and pepper. → Cover and simmer for 10 minutes or until zucchini is tender. → Add mushrooms and cook briefly, until the liquid evaporates. → Remove from heat. → Place in a small baking dish. → Cover with mozzarella cheese. → Bake for 10 minutes or until cheese is bubbly. → Serve warm. → you may serve with a *Baked Chicken Breast with Rosemary*.

see browning
see sautéing
see gratinéing

SALAD DRESSINGS AND SAUCES

1. PEPPER OIL

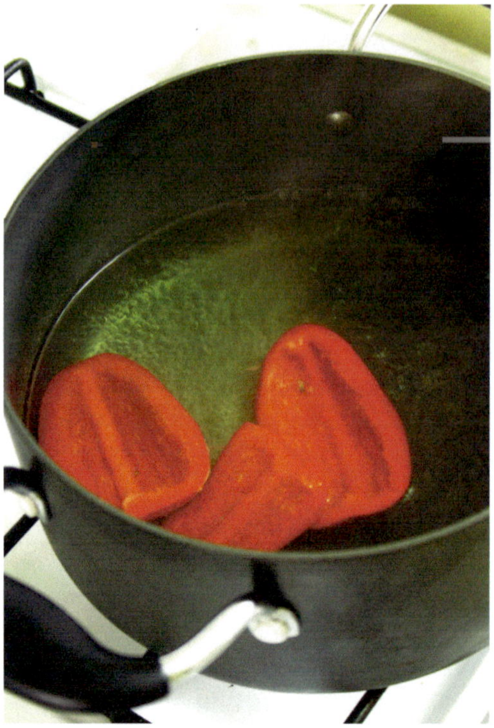

Serving amount: ½ cup
Preparation time: 10 minutes
Degree of difficulty: 3

Prepare the day before

1	PEPPER OIL (½ cup)			
	Ingredients for 4 to 6 portions	Equivalences		Calories
■	2 medium sized bell pepper (the color you prefer)			41.60
■	¼ cup extra virgin olive or avocado oil *			561.95
■	a pinch of salt and pepper			0.40
*	or any other gourmet oil of your choice	Total Calories		603.95

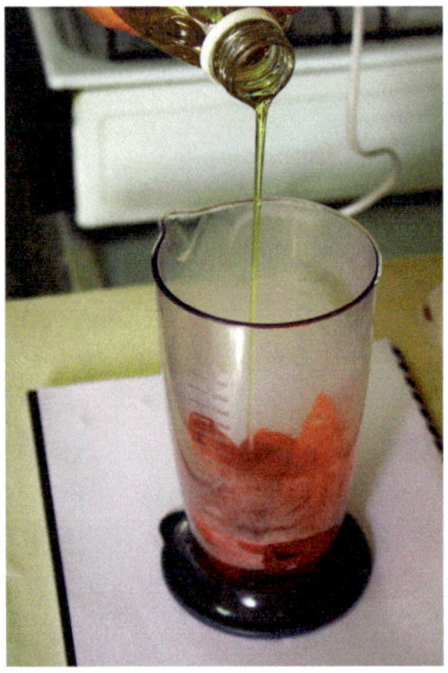

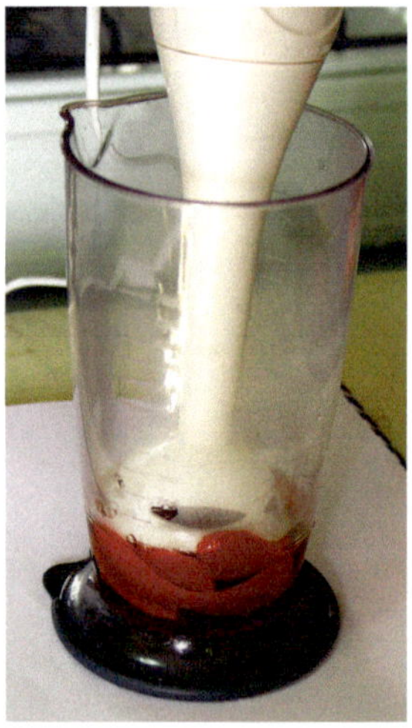

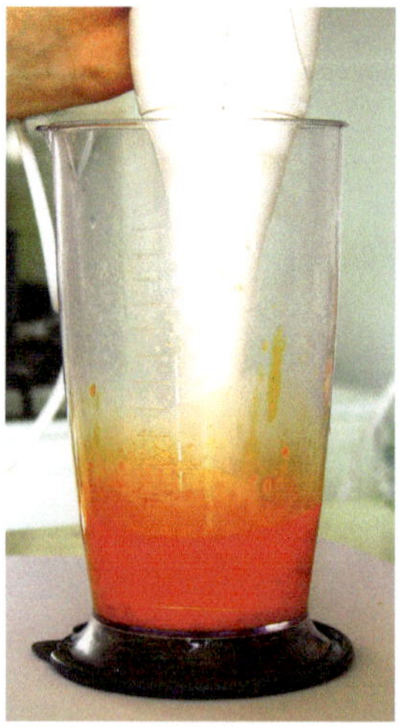

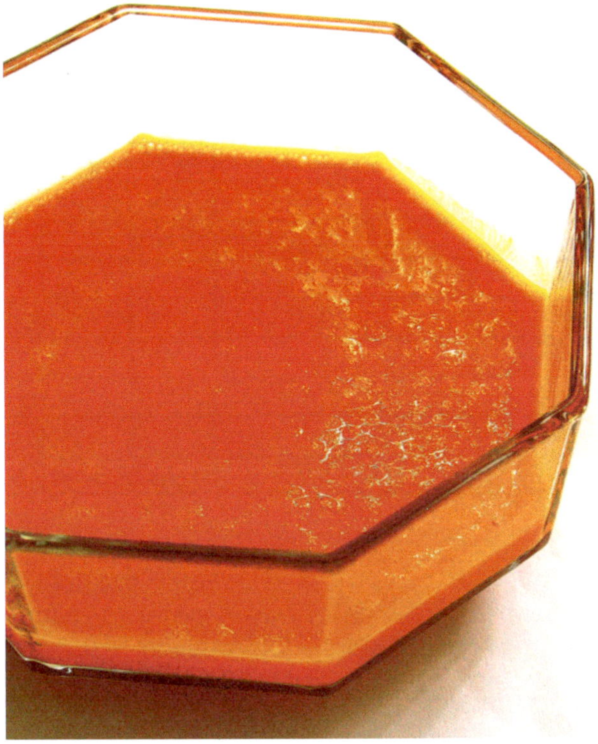

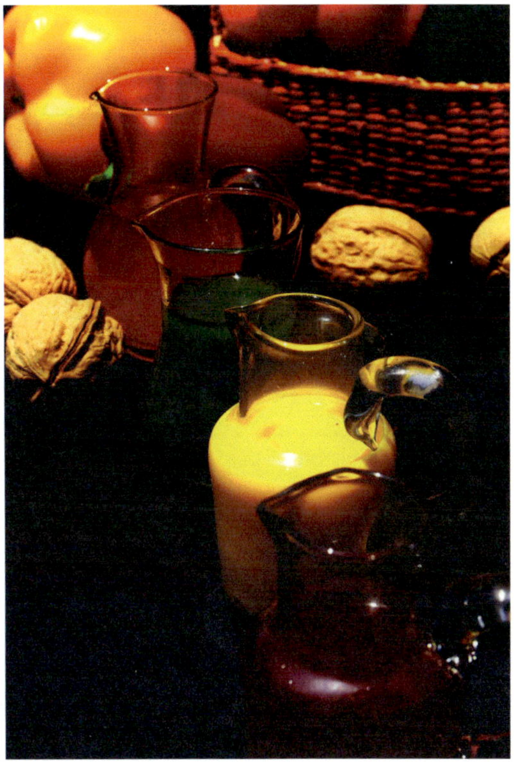

→ Blanch cut, peeled and seeded peppers. → Drain. → Blend pepper with oil. → Strain. → Pour in to a bowl and let stand in refrigerator overnight. → Next day, solids will separate from liquids. → Separate the oil form the peppers. → Use only the oil.

see blanching vegetables

The concentrated color of the used pepper which combined with oil gives gourmet foods new pleasant flavors, aromas and nuances.

Note: We recommend preparing small quantities, as pepper oil stays fresh for only 7 days when refrigerated.

Green peppers are a little bitter, while yellow, orange and especially red, are sweeter.

2. LEMON DRESSING

Serving amount: ¼ cup, 2- 4 portions
Preparation time: 5 minutes
Degree of difficulty: 1

2	LEMON DRESSING (¼ cup)			
	Ingredients for 2 to 4 portions	**Equivalences**		**Calories**
▪	1 tablespoons lemon juice, or the amount you wish	½	tbs.	1.60
▪	3 tablespoons extra virgin olive or avocado oil *			402.00
▪	¼ teaspoon powdered oregano			0.00
▪	¼ teaspoon splenda or			0.00
	¼ teaspoon brown sugar			5.00
▪	½ tablespoon low sodium soy sauce			5.00
▪	a pinch of pepper			0.40
*	or any other gourmet oil of your choice	**Total Calories**		**414.00**

→ Place in a bowl the lemon juice, olive or avocado oil, soy, oregano and pepper. → Season with salt and pepper. → Add ¼ teaspoon splenda or brown sugar to reduce acidity. → Mix well with a wire whisk. → Serve immediately. → Discard any remaining dressing.

3. HOMEMADE MAYONNAISE

Serving amount: 1 ¼ cup, 10- 12 portions
Preparation time: 10 minutes
Degree of difficulty: 2

3	HOMEMADE MAYONNAISE (1¼ cup)			
	Ingredients for 10 to 12 portions	Equivalences		Calories
▪	1 egg, preferably Omega-3			90.00
▪	1 cup extra virgin olive or avocado oil *			2247.80
▪	¼ teaspoon mustard			0.00
▪	½ tablespoon lemon juice			0.80
▪	a pinch of salt and pepper			0.40
*	or any other gourmet oil of your choice	Total Calories		**2339.00**

→ Pour ¼ cup oil into a blender. → Add all ingredients and blend for 10 seconds. → Continue blending and gradually add the remaining oil until it thickens. → Season with salt and pepper. → Pour into a airtight container and refrigerate. → Keeps for up to 5 days.

4. HOMEMADE MAYONNAISE WITH CURRY

Serving amount: 1 ¼ cup, 10-12 portions
Preparation time: 11 minutes
Degree of difficulty: 2

4	HOMEMADE MAYONNAISE WITH CURRY (1¼ cup)			
	Ingredients for 10 to 12 portions	Equivalences		Calories
▪	1 egg, preferably Omega-3 egg			90.00
▪	1 cup extra virgin olive or avocado oil*			2247.80
▪	1 ½ teaspoon curry			0.00
▪	¼ teaspoon mustard			0.00
▪	½ tablespoon lemon juice, or the amount you wish			0.80
▪	a pinch of salt and pepper			0.40
*	or any other gourmet oil of your choice	Total Calories		**2339.00**

→ Pour ¼ cup oil into a blender. → Add all ingredients and blend for 10 seconds. → Continue blending and gradually add the remaining oil until thickened. → Season with salt and pepper. → Pour into an airtight container and refrigerate. → Keeps for up to 5 days.

5. BASIC TOMATO SAUCE

Serving amount: ¾ cup, 2 portions
Preparation time: 30 minutes
Degree of difficulty: 3

5	**BASIC TOMATO SAUCE (¾ cup)**			
	Ingredients for 2 portions	**Equivalences**		**Calories**
▪	1 cup tomatoes peeled, seeded and chopped			27.00
▪	1 bay leaf			0.00
▪	1 teaspoon extra-virgin olive or avocado oil			134.00
▪	½ cup lean ground chicken (optional)	125 g	4.3 oz	67.40
▪	1 teaspoon crushed garlic			2.30
▪	½ cup hot water			0.00
▪	a pinch of salt and pepper			0.40
		Total Calories		**231.10**

→ Heat oil in a non-stick frying pan. → Add garlic and brown slightly. → Add tomatoes and bay leaf. → Simmer until tomato reduces to a sauce. → Stir and reduce sauce for 10 more minutes. → Add ½ cup of hot water. → Stir sauce until it thickened. → Discard bay leaf and season with salt and pepper. → Remove sauce from heat and serve warm. → We recommend serving 3 tablespoons per ½ cup of cooked pasta per person. → Freeze remaining sauce when cool. → Store it in an airtight container for up to 30 days.

With ground meat:

→ After browning garlic add ½ cup of ground chicken. → Sauté slightly. → Follow original recipe instructions. → We recommend serving the sauce with cooked vegetables. → Freeze remaining sauce when cool. → Store in an airtight container for up to 30 days.

see peeling raw tomatoes
see browning
see reducing liquids
see sautéing

6. SWEET AND SOUR VINAIGRETTE

Serving amount: ¾ cup, 6-8 portions
Preparation time: 10 minutes
Degree of difficulty: 2

6	SWEET AND SOUR VINAIGRETTE (¾ cup)			
	Ingredients for 6 to 8 portions	**Equivalences**		**Calories**
▪	1 egg yolk, preferably omega-3 egg			50.80
▪	2 tablespoons balsamic vinegar (or apple cider vinegar for a milder flavor)			2.30
▪	1 tablespoon honey			43.20
▪	½ cup extra-virgin olive or avocado oil *			1123.90
*	or any other gourmet oil of your choice	**Total Calories**		**1220.20**

→ Place egg yolks and oil in a bowl. → Mix well with a wire whisk. → Add vinegar and honey. → Beat and mix well. → Keep in remainder the rest refrigerated for up to 3 days.

7. MUSTARD VINAIGRETTE

Serving amount: ¼ cup, 2-4 portions
Preparation time: 5 minutes
Degree of difficulty: 2

7	MUSTARD VINAIGRETTE (¼ cup)			
	Ingredients for 2 to 4 portions	**Equivalences**		**Calories**
▪	½ tablespoon apple cider vinegar			0.30
▪	1 ½ tablespoons extra virgin olive or avocado oil*			201.00
▪	1 tablespoon Dijon mustard			0.00
▪	a pinch of salt and pepper			0.40
*	or any other gourmet oil of your choice	**Total Calories**		**201.70**

→ Place all ingredients into a small mixing bowl. → Mix well with a wire whisk. → Refrigerate remaining vinaigrette for up to 3 days.

DESSERTS AND DRINKS

1. SWEET POTATO A L'ORANGE

Chef Marcelo Portuondo's recipe

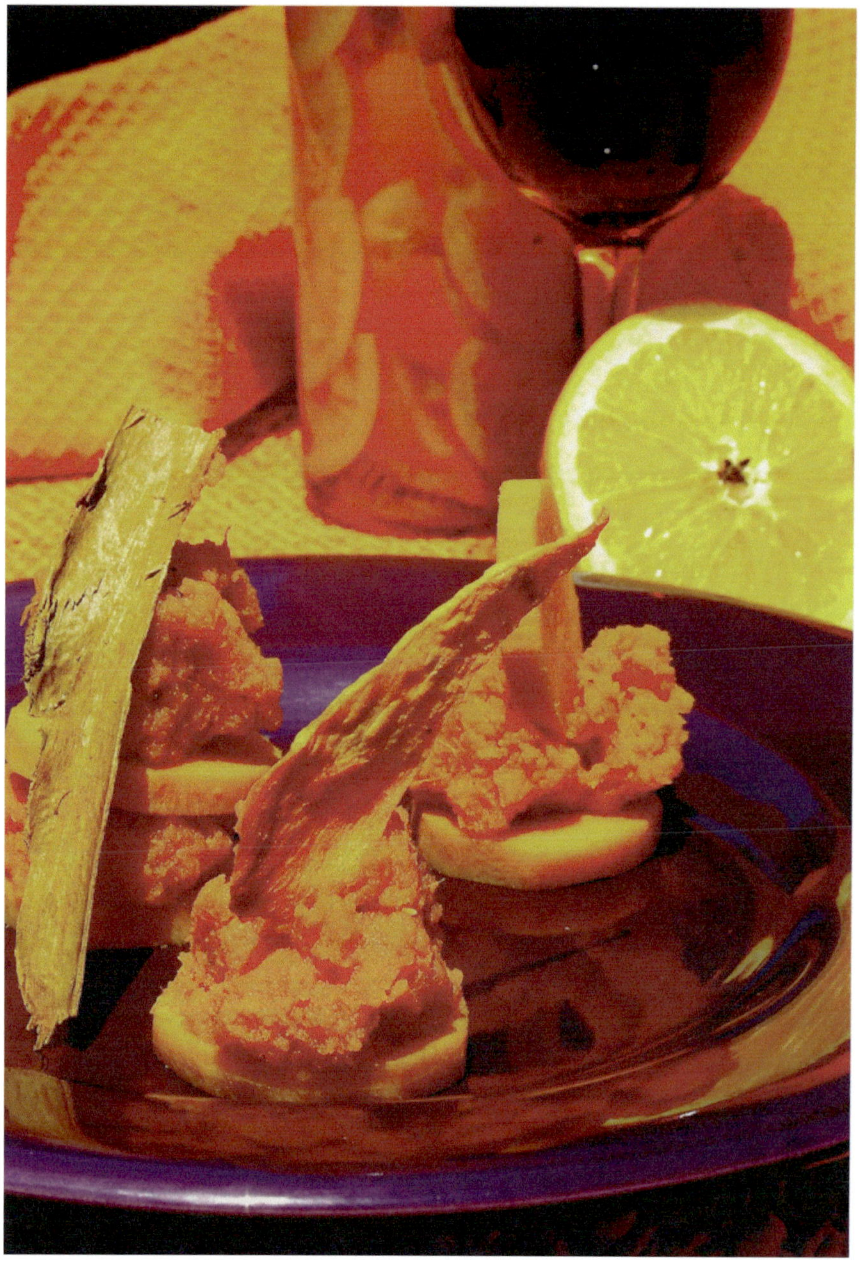

Serves 2
Preparation time: 1 hour, 40 minutes
Degree of difficulty: 2

1	SWEET POTATO A L'ORANGE			
	Ingredients for 2 portions	**Equivalences**		**Calories**
▪	1 medium sized sweet potato			90.80
▪	1 teaspoon butter			37.00
▪	3 cinnamon sticks			0.00
▪	juice of 1 orange	¼	cup	73.00
▪	2 orange slices, round			18.25
▪	¼ teaspoon orange zest, washed and grated orange rid			0.00
▪	1 tablespoons splenda or			0.00
	1 teaspoon brown sugar (optional)			20.00
▪	1 tablespoon Port wine (optional)			23.55
▪	a pinch of salt and pepper			0.40
		Total Calories		**263.00**

Preheat oven to 350º F – 180º C

To prepare sweet potato:

→ Wash and stuff sweet potato with 2 cinnamon sticks. → Wrap sweet potato with orange slices in aluminum foil. → Bake in oven on a cookie sheet for 1 ½ hours or until soft to touch. → Remove from oven. → Peel sweet potato while still warm. → Press pulp with a tablespoon through a strainer until obtaining a creamy, lump free purée. → Set aside.

To prepare syrup:

→ Heat splenda or brown sugar, orange juice, a cinnamon stick and a spoonful of port (optional) wine in a small sauce pan. → Stir constantly with a wooden spoon for about 5 minutes, until it forms a (light) syrup. → Add the mashed sweet potatoes and mix well. → Check the sweetness, remove from heat and add butter. → This flavorful purée is served as dessert or as an accompaniment to turkey, chicken or pork.

Note: The presentation of the recipe suggests placing the purée over a round slice of cooked sweet potato. The garnish placed on the purée is a slice of crunchy sweet potato. (Bake a thin slice of raw sweet potato in a microwave oven at maximum temperature for 3 minutes)

See stuffing sweet potatoes

2. ASSORTED FRUIT WITH YOGURT, HONEY AND SESAME

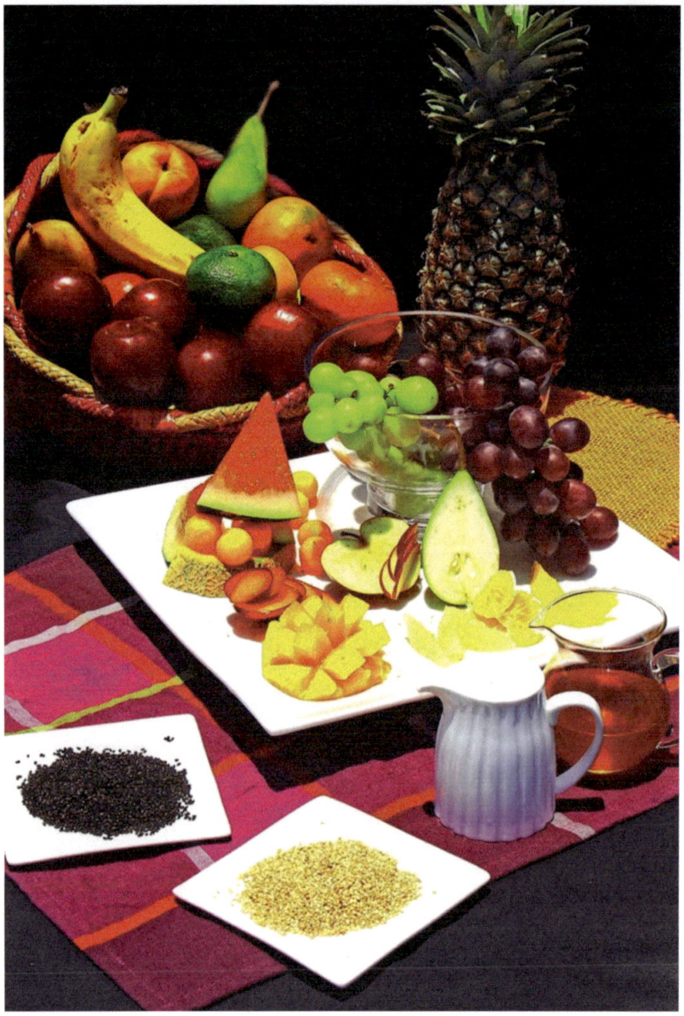

Serves 1
Preparation time: 10 minutes
Degree of difficulty: 1

2	ASSORTED FRUITS WITH YOGURT, HONEY AND ASSORTED SEEDS			
	Suggested accompaniments	Equivalences		Calories
■	2 tablespoons fat free plain yogurt	¼	cup	40.00
■	1 tablespoon honey			43.21
■	½ teaspoon toasted sesame seeds or			44.80
	5 toasted almonds			54.00
■	5 raisins or			13.00
	2 cherries			40.00
■	1 tablespoon lemon juice* (optional)			1.60
*	for the Assorted Fruits	Total Calories		**236.61**

Combinations of suggested fruits (per person)

	1. Assorted Fruits			
	Combinations of suggested fruits (per person)	**Equivalences**		**Calories**
▪	½ banana, cut into 3 ½ inch slices			42.60
▪	8 strawberries			17.20
▪	½ red apple peeled and cut into 3 slices			23.00
		Total Calories		**82.80**

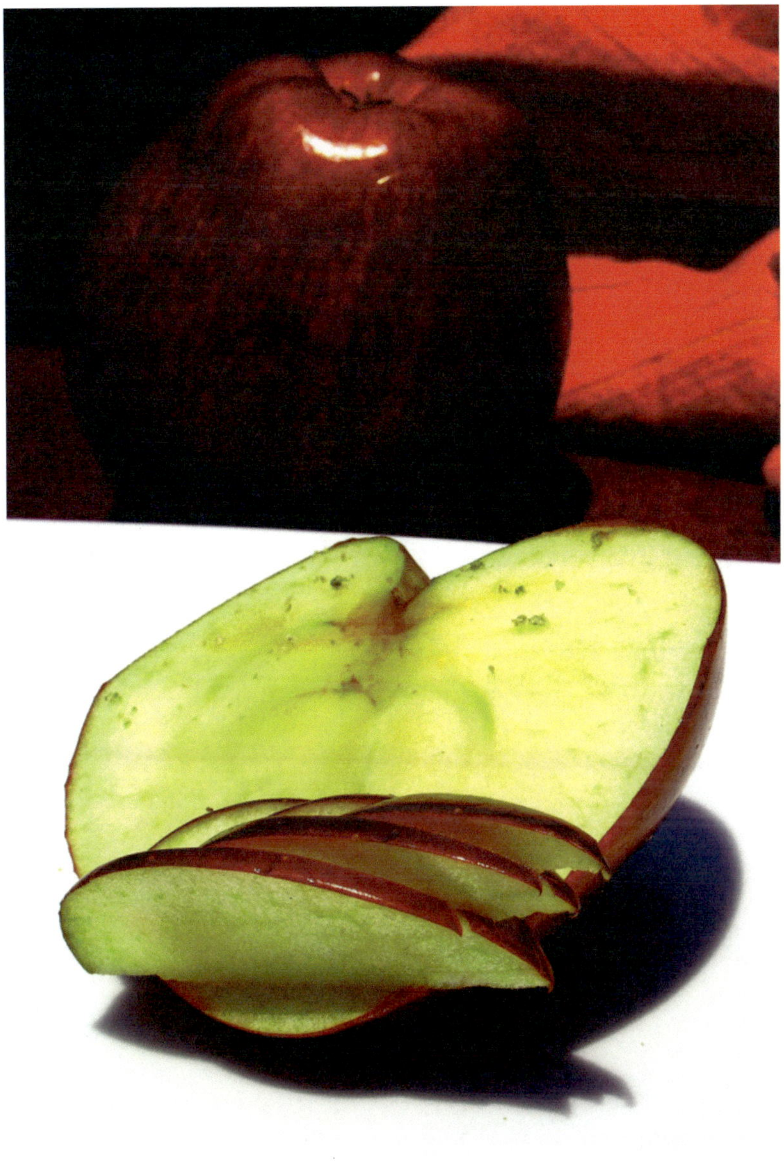

	2. Sliced citrus			
	Combinations of suggested fruits (per person)	**Equivalences**		**Calories**
▪	½ tangerine (4 slices)			18.50
▪	½ grapefruit (4 slices)			13.80
▪	½ cup papaya, chopped			13.30
		Total Calories		**45.60**

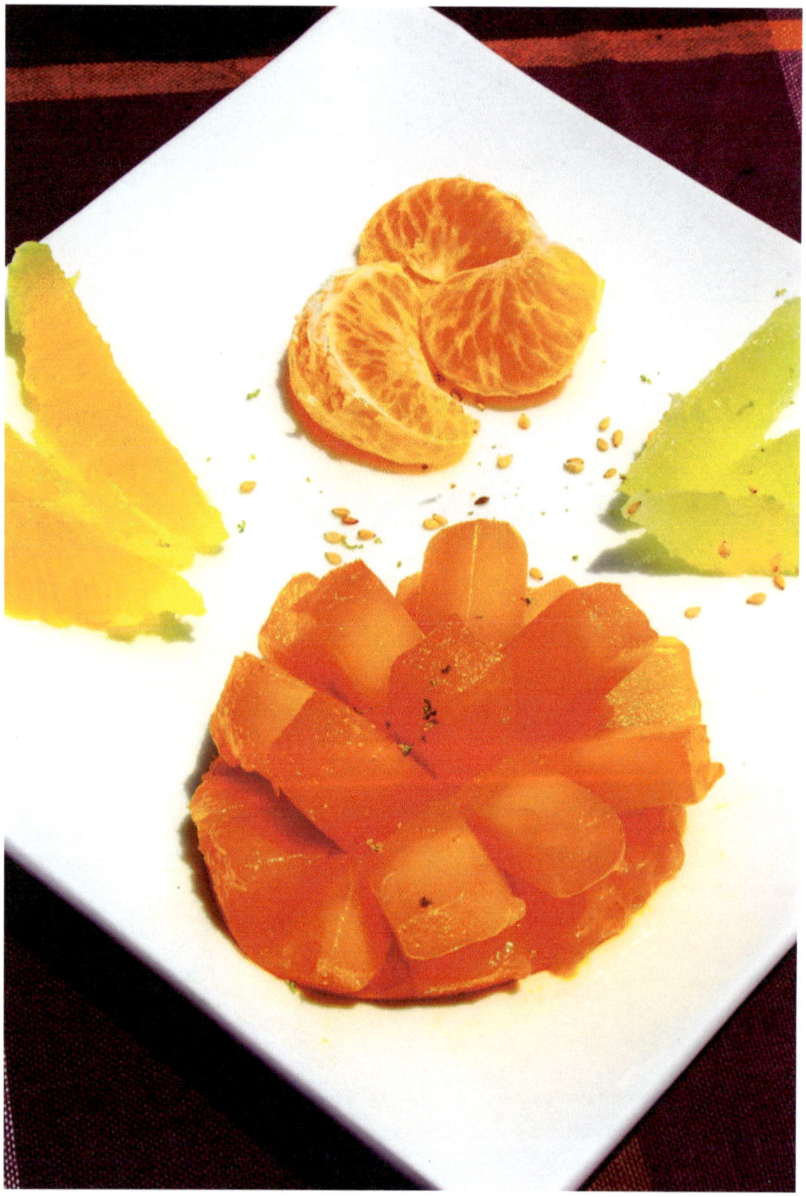

	3. Berries of the forest (cultivated in your region)			
	Combinations of suggested fruits (per person)	**Equivalences**		**Calories**
▪	5 strawberries (50 g)			17.20
▪	8 raspberries			19.50
▪	½ pear or 4 blackberries			23.20 17.50
		Total Calories		**77.40**

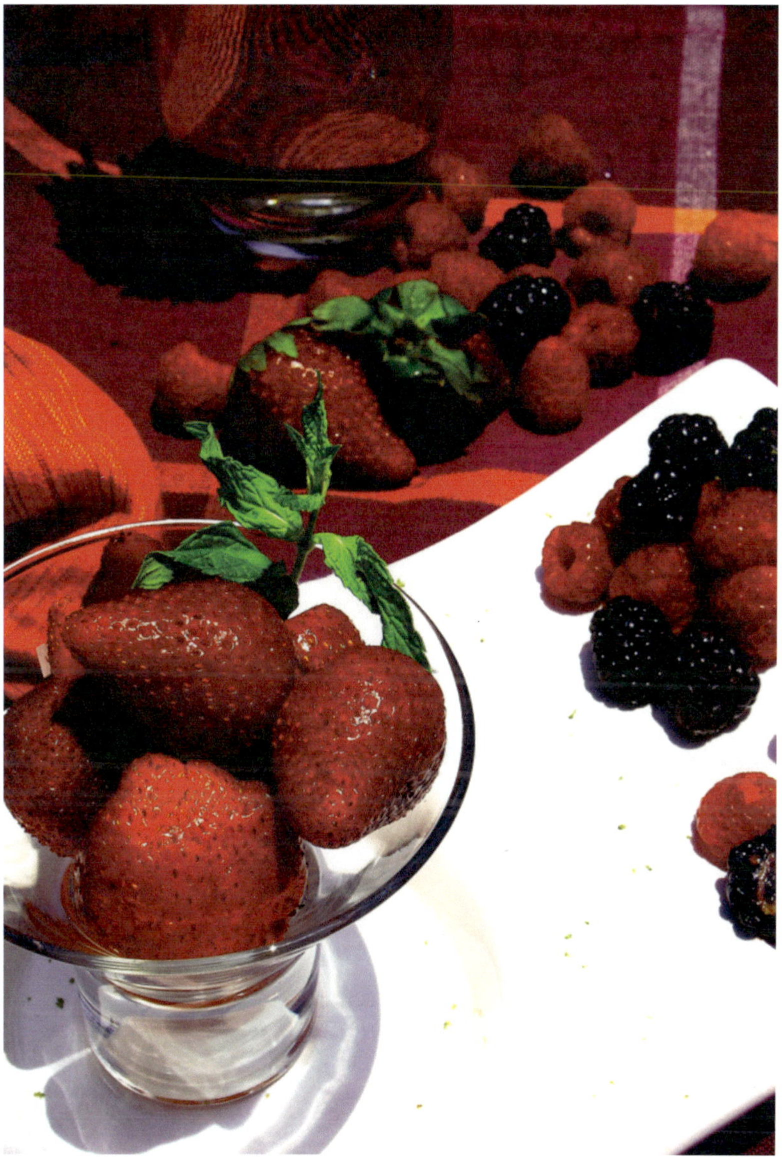

	4. Water fruits			
Combinations of suggested fruits (per person)		Equivalences		Calories
▪	4 small melon balls			26.20
▪	4 small watermelon balls			10.14
▪	1 plum			22.50
		Total Calories		**58.84**

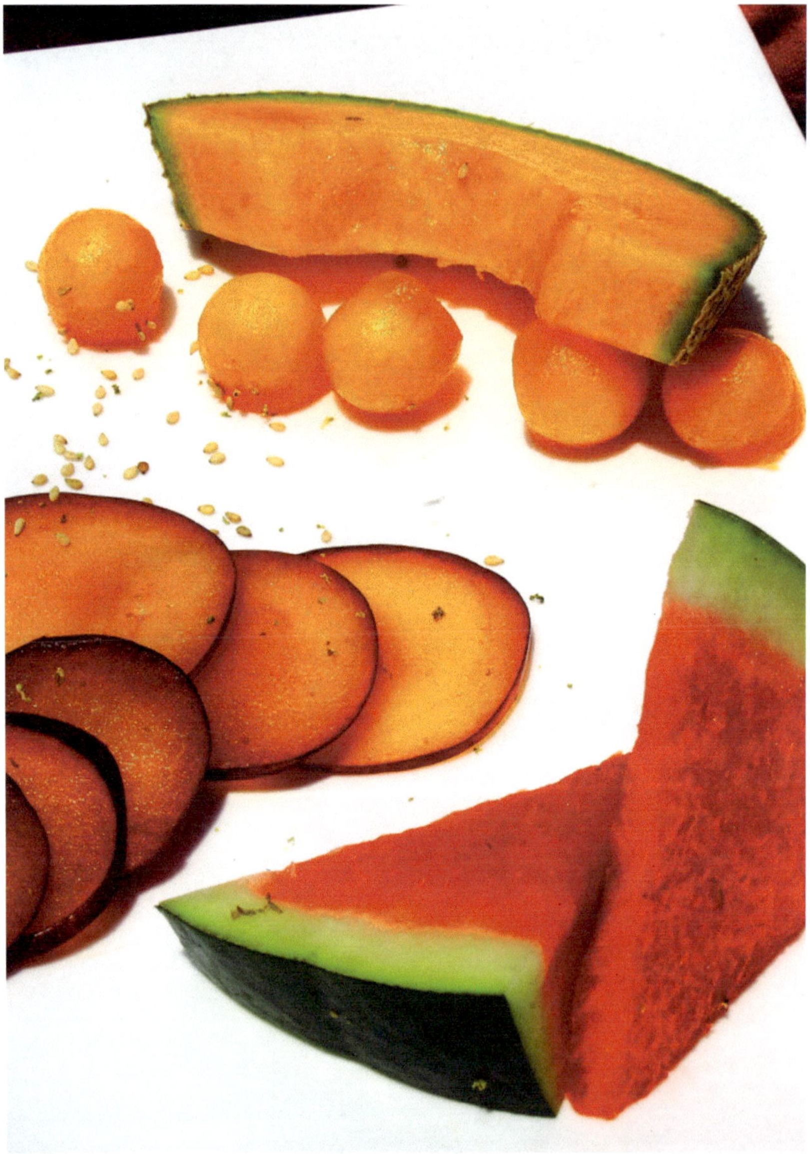

5. Tri-color grapes

	Combinations of suggested fruits (per person)	Equivalences		Calories
▪	15 white grapes			18.00
▪	15 red grapes			20.00
▪	15 black grapes			20.00
		Total Calories		**58.00**

6. Tropical flavor

	Combinations of suggested fruits (per person)	Equivalences		Calories
▪	½ small mango			30.00
		Total Calories		**30.00**

7. Tropical touch

	Combinations of suggested fruits (per person)	Equivalences		Calories
▪	3 slices pineapple			23.00
		Total Calories		**23.00**

→ Place sliced fruits in an individual fruit bowl. → Add yogurt. → Cover with honey and sprinkle seeds on top. → Serve immediately.

Note: → If fruits are prepared in advance, drizzle them with lemon juice to prevent oxidation. → Keep refrigerated in an airtight container. → Add accompaniments before serving.

See toasting sesame seeds
See peeling and toasting almonds

3. ORANGE, CINNAMON AND CLOVE GELATIN

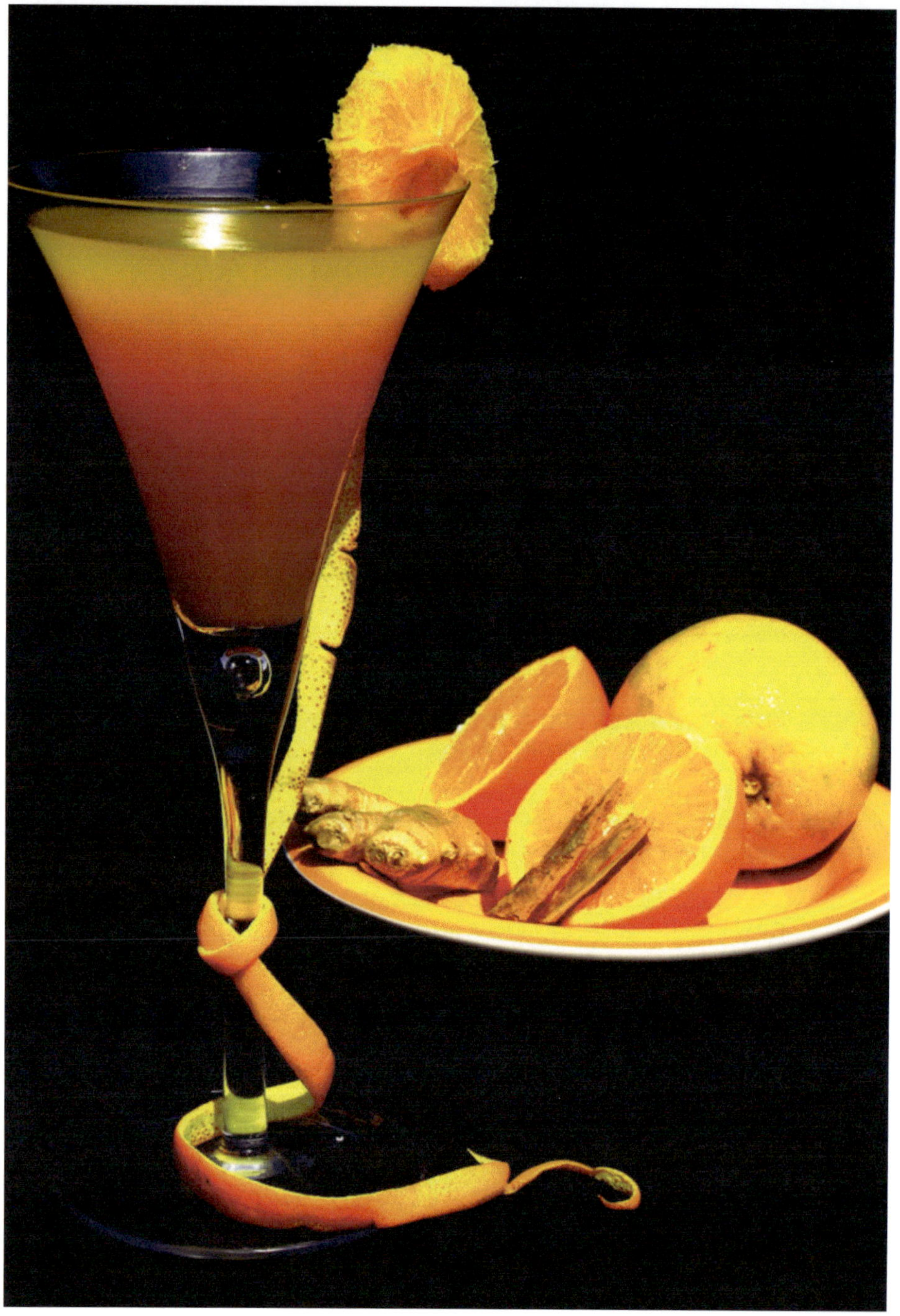

Serves 2
Preparation time: 20 minutes
Refrigeration time: 1-2 hours
Degree of difficulty: 2

3	ORANGE, CINNAMON AND CLOVE GELATIN			
	Ingredients for 2 portions	**Equivalences**		**Calories**
■	1 sugar free orange gelatin package 3 oz.			50.50
■	½ cup boiling water			0.00
■	1½ cup sweet orange juice, undiluted			137.10
■	2 tablespoons splenda * or			0.00
	1 tablespoon brown sugar (optional)			60.00
■	1 clove			0.00
■	1 small slice peeled fresh ginger (optional)			0.00
■	2 cinnamon sticks			0.00
*	depending on the sweetness of orange juice	**Total Calories**		**247.60**

→ Dissolve gelatin in 1 cup boiling water. → Then add 1 cup of cold water. → Stir and set aside. → Place the orange juice, cinnamon, clove and slice of ginger in a medium sized pan over low heat. → Stir constantly with a wooden spoon. → Reduce the liquid stirring for about 15 minutes. → Avoid boiling. → Remove from heat. → Discard the cinnamon, ginger and cloves. → Add to preparation the gelatin dissolved beforehand cool. → Mix well and pour the liquid into tall glasses. → Refrigerate for 1 or 2 hours or until gelatin is solid. → Garnish with pulp and orange peel. → Serve chilled.

Note: Ginger must be soft and fresh, otherwise it can give a bitter taste to the preparation.

see reducing liquids

4. STRAWBERRY FRAPPÉ JUICE

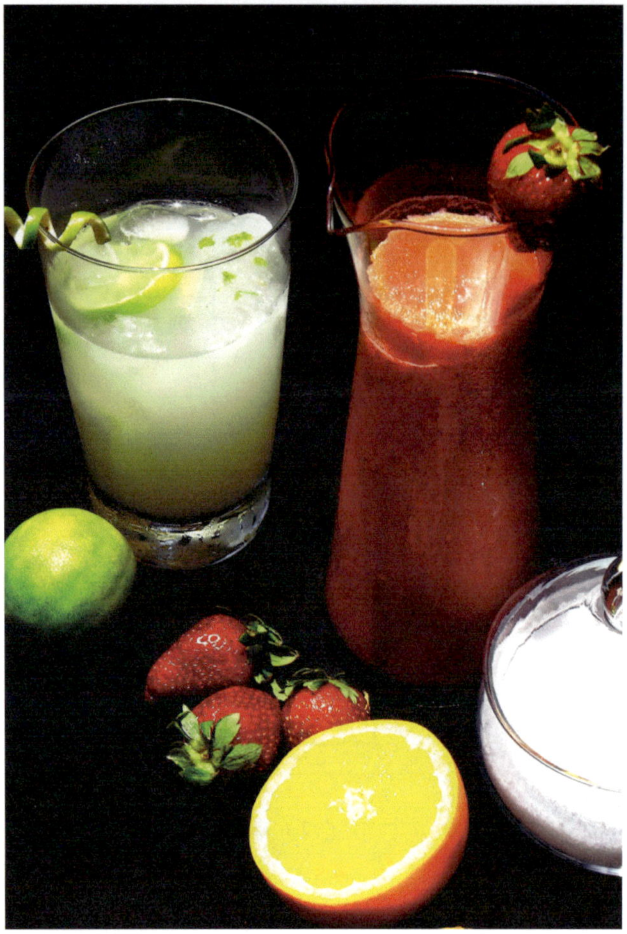

Serves 2
Preparation time: 5 minutes
Degree of difficulty: 1

4	STRAWBERRY FRAPPÉ			
	Ingredients for 2 glasses	**Equivalences**		**Calories**
▪	2 cups medium sized strawberries, washed and halved			78.00
▪	2 whole strawberries for garnish			15.60
▪	½ cup orange juice			45.70
▪	3 tablespoons splenda or			0.00
	1 tablespoon brown sugar			60.00
▪	4 medium sized ice cubes (equivalent to ½ cup water)			0.00
		Total Calories		**199.30**

→ Blend strawberries and orange juice. → Add ice and continue blending. → Add brown sugar or splenda and finish blending. → Serve in ice cream cups, or tall parfait glasses. → Garnish with a whole strawberry.

5. FROZEN LEMONADE

Serves 1
Preparation time: 5 minutes
Degree of difficulty: 1

5	FROZEN LEMONADE			
	Ingredients for 1 glass	**Equivalences**		**Calories**
▪	2 tablespoons lemon juice, or the amount desired	2	tbs.	3.20
▪	grated lemon zest, grated rind *			0.00
▪	3 tablespoons splenda or amount desired, or			0.00
	1 tablespoon brown sugar			60.00
▪	1 lemon slice for garnish (optional)			0.00
▪	8 medium-sized ice cubes (1 cup of water or the amount you wish)			0.00
		Total Calories		**63.20**

→ Squeeze 4 lemons and pour juice into blender. → Add brown sugar or splenda and blend well. → Add the ice and finish blending. → Serve in sorbet dish or tall glass. → Garnish with the peel, grated lemon and a lemon slice.

6. HOT OR ICED GREEN TEA WITH LEMON

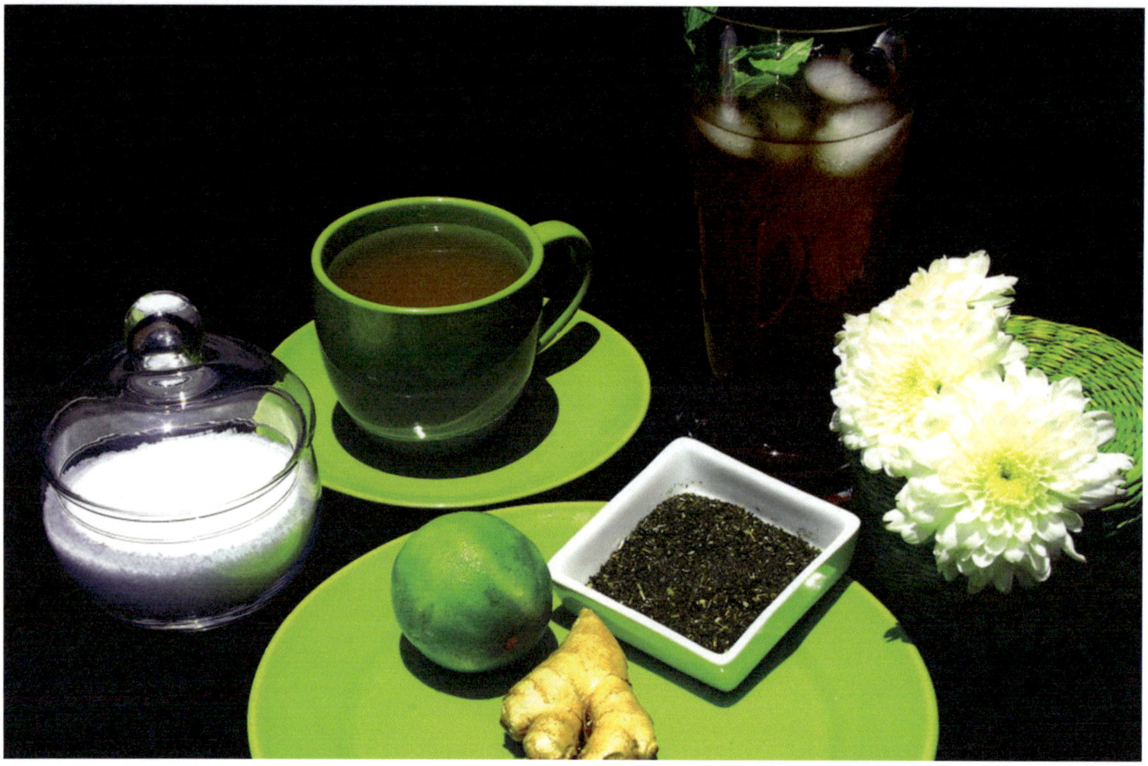

Serving amount:1 cup
Preparation time for hot green tea: 7 minutes
Preparation time for iced green tea: 30 minutes
Degree of difficulty: 1

6	HOT OR ICED GREEN TEA WITH LEMON			
	Ingredients for 1 cup	**Equivalences**		**Calories**
▪	1 green tea bag			0.00
▪	½ tablespoon lemon juice, or the amount desired			0.80
▪	¼ teaspoon small piece lemon zest			0.00
▪	2 or 3 teaspoon splenda or the amount you wish, or			0.00
	1 teaspoon brown sugar (optional)			20.00
▪	1 cup boiling water			0.00
		Total Calories		**20.80**

Hot tea:

→ Boil a cup of water. → Remove from heat. → Allow to cool for 3 minutes. → Place the green tea bag in an empty cup. → Add hot water and slice of lemon peel. → Cover and steep for 3 minutes. → Remove the bag and the piece of lemon peel. → Serve hot. → Add splenda or brown sugar and stir well before drinking.

Iced tea:

→ Follow hot green tea recipe instructions. → Allow it to cool and refrigerate. → Serve in a tall glass. →

Note: If you wish, you can add crushed ice.

7. HOT OR ICED GREEN TEA WITH MINT AND GINGER

Serving amount:1 cup
Preparation time for hot green tea: 7 minutes
Preparation time for iced green tea: 30 minutes
Degree of difficulty: 2

7	HOT OR ICED GREEN TEA WITH MINT AND GINGER			
	Ingredients for 1 cup	**Equivalences**		**Calories**
▪	1 green tea bag for infusion			0.00
▪	2 leaves or 1 sprig of fresh mint			0.00
▪	1 teaspoons splenda or			0.00
	1 teaspoon brown sugar (optional)			20.00
▪	1 small slice fresh ginger, peeled			0.00
▪	1 cup boiling water			0.00
		Total Calories		**20.00**

Hot tea:

→ Boil a cup of water. → Remove from heat. → Allow to cool for 3 minutes. → Place the green tea bag in an empty cup. → Add hot water, mint and ginger. → Cover end steep for 3 minutes. → Remove the bag, ginger and mint. → Serve hot. → Add splenda or brown sugar and stir well before drinking.

Iced tea:

→ Follow Hot Green Tea recipe instructions above. → Remove the tea bag, ginger and mint. → Allow it to cool and refrigerate. → Serve in a tall glass. → Add brown sugar or splenda and mix well. → Garnish with a mint leaf.

Note: If you wish, you can add crushed ice.

Blanching vegetables technique

This procedure ensures a firm texture "al dente", an intense color and nice flavor. Vitamin and mineral content is preserved. Vegetables are cooked according to the chart and then quickly plunged into ice water for no more than one minute.

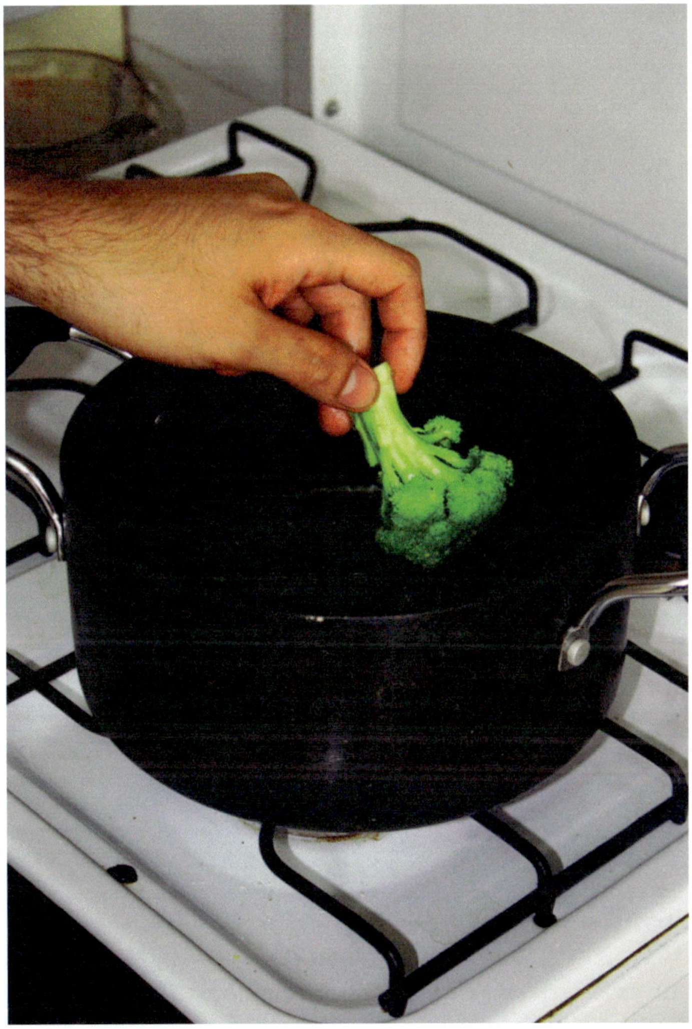

Broccoli is being used as an example to explain the procedure. For other vegetables used in recipes, see cooking times table for Blanching Vegetables.

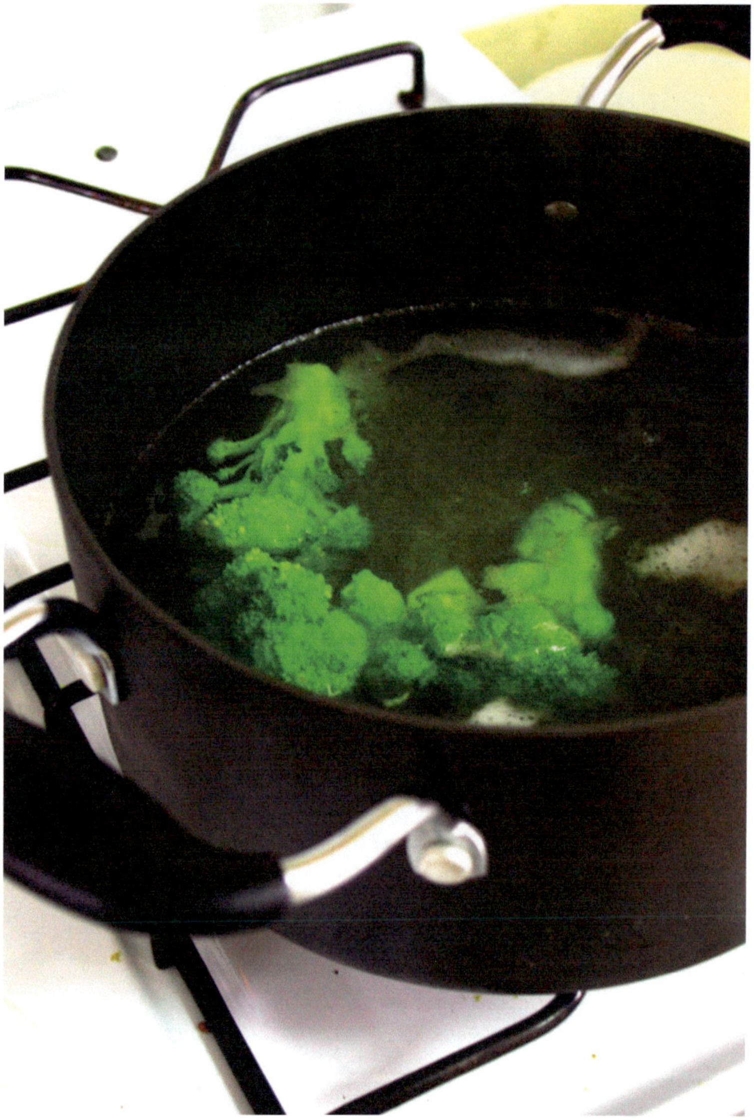

→ Into a bowl pour 3 cups of cold water and approximately 10 ice cubes. → Set aside. → Wash vegetables well. → Cut broccoli florets in the same size. → Boil 3 cups water in medium pan. → Wait until you have a rolling boil. → Add ½ teaspoon of salt and stir. → Drop in vegetables and cook *al dente,* for no more 3 minutes. → Remove pan from heat and pour off hot water. → To stop cooking, quickly plunge the vegetables in the bowl of ice and cold water. → Remove after one minute. → Drain well and serve.

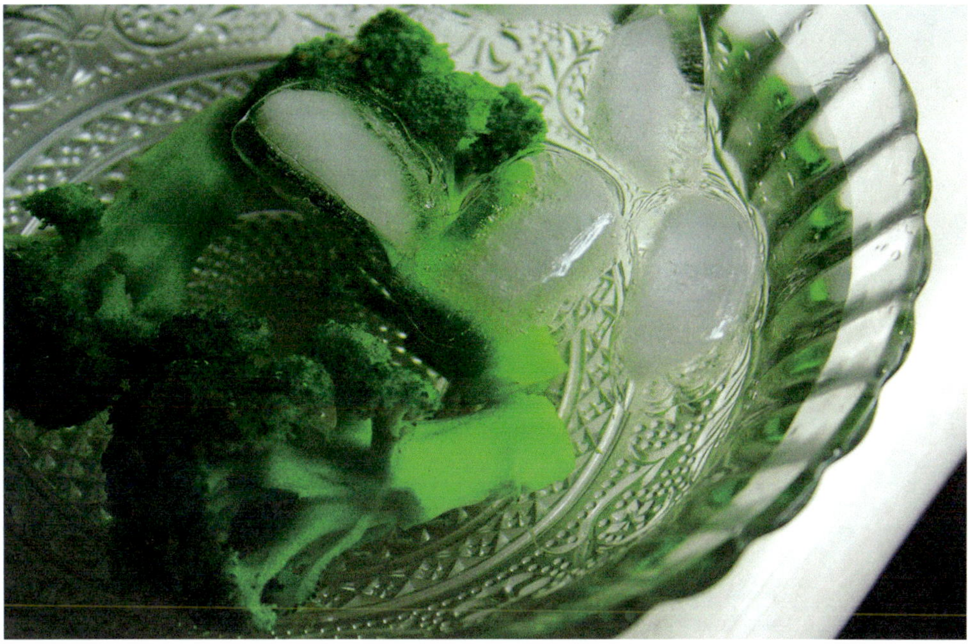

Culinary note: we suggest blanching vegetables right before serving to avoid losing its texture.

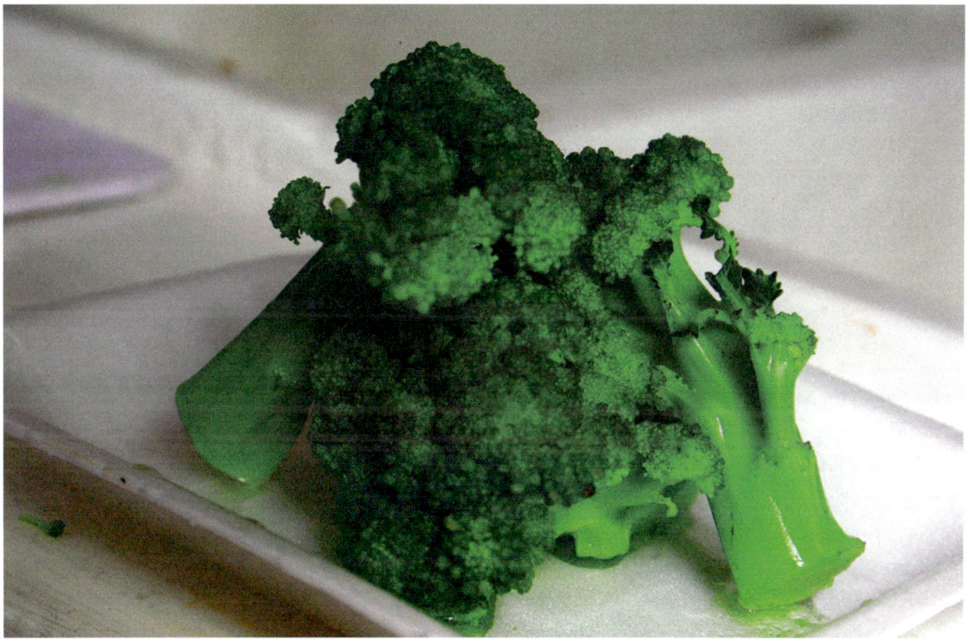

Reusing the blanching water

Blanch different types of vegetables with ease. Blanch one vegetable after the other. Start with vegetables that need less cooking time.

Example: broccoli and carrots. → Cook the broccoli for 3 minutes. → Remove with slotted spoon from pot. → Plunge in ice water. → Remove to serving dish. → Repeat with carrots.

If you want to obtain a further benefit of the water from blanching of vegetables, reuse it to cook skinless, chicken breasts. The concentrated broth will have a pleasant taste and will contain nutrients from the vegetables.

Cooking Times Table for Blanching Vegetables

Before blanching vegetables, we recommend selecting or cutting them the same size. The thickness, the cut and the vegetable chosen, will determine its cooking time.

1 cup	Beetroot, whole	15	minutes
1 cup	Brussels Sprouts, whole	9	minutes
1 cup	Baby corn	7	minutes
1 cup	Zucchini	5	minutes
1 cup	Okra [1]	4	minutes
1 cup	Carrots, cut into medium pieces	3	and a half minutes
1 cup	Peppers, chopped, seeded	3	and a half minutes
1 cup	Young baby cabbage	3	minutes
1 cup	Cauliflower florets	3	minutes
1 cup	Broccoli florets	3	minutes
1 cup	Baby carrots	3	minutes
1 cup	Green beans	2	and a half minutes
1 cup	Asparagus, small, medium or large [2]	2	minutes
1 cup	Peas, common or big [3]	1	minute
1 cup	Spinach [4]	30	seconds
1 cup	Chinese Bean [4]	20	seconds

Additional information of some vegetables included in the Table:

1 **Okra**: (okra) is a leguminous plant containing mucilage. The mucilage is an organic compound of bitter taste, with a viscous consistency like glue. To avoid releasing of the mucilaginous juice during blanching, we recommend the following steps: → Boil 3 cups of water in a medium pot. → Add a tablespoon of white vinegar. → Wash okra and boil for 4 minutes. → Remove okra with a slotted spoon and plunge in ice water for 1 minute. → Remove and drain well. → Dress with a squeeze of lemon before serving.

2 **Asparagus of different size and thickness**. → Make 3 cups of ice water in a medium size bowl. → Set aside. → Wash and sort the asparagus according to size. → Snap off and discard the though ends. → Boil 3 cups of water in a medium size bowl.→ Add ½ teaspoon of salt and stir. → Introduce the largest asparagus and cook for 2 minutes. → Then, add the smaller ones and cook for 2 minutes. → Remove pot form heat. → Quickly remove asparagus with tongs. → Plunge for 1 minute in the ice water. → Allow drying briefly on absorbent paper towels. → Serve right away to prevent vegetables from becoming wilted. XXX

Culinary Note: We recommend selecting asparagus the same size and thickness for a uniform cooking time.

3 **Peas**: it is preferable to use raw and small green peas to prevent wrinkling. Do not blanch, they and incorporated at the end of the recipes, cook quickly and remain tender.

4 **Mung Bean sprouts and Spinach**: blanch only 20 to 30 seconds, respectively.

→ Make 3 cups of ice water with 10 ice cubes in a bowl. → Set aside. → Arrange the mung beans or spinach leaves in a colander and wash thoroughly. → Place the colander in the sink. → Pour over sprouts or spinach. a steady stream of boiling water for the time indicated. → (You can use the teapot with boiling water.) → Quickly remove from strainer with tongs. → Remove the blanched vegetables and drain in colander. → Allow drying briefly on absorbent paper towels. → Use right away to prevent vegetables from becoming wilted.

Medical Reasons to Dialyze Vegetables:

In our book recipes we use the "**blanching**" technique for cooking many of the vegetables. However, some people are advised to not consume foods with naturally occurring salt or minerals (such as dialysis patients) and it is recommended that another process called dialyzing is used. This process will remove these unwanted, natural ingredients. Broccoli is used to demonstrate the basics of this technique.

Dialyzing vegetables

→ Wash the broccoli thoroughly. → Cut into florets of the same size. → In a medium sized pan, bring 3 cups of water (without salt) to a boil. → Gently place the vegetables into the water bath and cook until tender (parboil), probably less than 5 minutes.→ Remove the pan from heat. Drain off the cooking water. Carefully pour through a colander place in the sink taking care not to scald yourself with the steam. → Serve immediately. → In more severe cases, it is required to **dialyze** the vegetables two or more times to more fully remove the salts and minerals. → The water used in each dialysis must be discarded.

Culinary note: To compensate the loss of nutrients, flavors and aromas, we recommend seasoning foods with gourmet oils and herbs.

Blanching and toasting almonds

Used in recipe: Spinach and Mushroom Salad in Soy Sauce

Preheat oven to 350º F or 180º C

Blanched and toasted almonds... → Add 3 cups of water to a medium sized pan. → Place over heat and bring to a boil. → Add the almonds and boil for 2 minutes. → Remove pan from heat and pour off hot water.→ To stop the cooking quickly plunge the almonds into a bowl with ice water for 1 minute. → Remove almonds from water and dry with a paper towel. → Peel the skin off by rubbing them gently with fingers. → Bake the almonds on a cookie sheet for 5 minutes or until lightly browned.

Culinary Note: Monitor the process to avoid overcooking. → To keep toasted almonds fresh, refrigerate in an airtight container for up to 6 months.

Pasta "al dente"

Used in recipes: Spaghetti with vegetables and olives
Macaroni with tofu and mushrooms

Al dente is an Italian term that is literally translated "to the tooth", meaning that the outside is cooked but the center has a bit of resistance to the bite, in other words, neither overcooked nor mushy. Traditionally al dente was used to describe the cooking stage of pasta but today it is increasingly applied to the cooking of vegetables and legumes. This technique helps to protect the vitamin content of foods and retains more of the natural flavors, especially when the products are fresh and of excellent quality.

Experts consider it the ideal way to cook pasta. They also recommend this "crunchy" consistency as the goal for cooked or blanched vegetables.

→ Bring 4 cups of water to a boil in a medium sized pan. → Add 1 tablespoon of salt and stir to dissolve. → Add 2 tablespoons of oil to prevent sticking of the pasta. → Slowly add 1 cup of pasta or noodles attempting to maintain the boil. → Stir gently and minimally to avoid breaking the noodles / pasta. → Cook for a few minutes (follow product instructions) until pasta is *al dente*. → Remove from heat. → Drain pasta in a colander. → Use as stated in the recipe.

To find out if the pasta is *"al dente"* remove a piece of pasta using a slotted spoon. Cut in half and check if it still has a thin center of raw pasta which will be of a slightly different color. This is seen very clearly in the case of the macaroni.

Medical note:
Pasta prepared "*al dente*" is slightly more difficult to digest than when more thoroughly cooked.

Medical note:
The pasta "*al dente*" is slightly more difficult to digest than when cooked.

Washing and cooking legumes al dente

Used in recipes: Chickpea and Sprout Salad
Lentils with Vegetables

Before preparing any dried legume (lentil, bean, pea) we recommend to pick through them looking for stones and ones that are broken or discolored. Wash in a strainer and discard the water.

Most legumes contain sugars that may cause flatulence (gas) and indigestion. To avoid this soak legumes for 4 hours in fresh water at room temperature. Discard the water which will have leeched off at least some of these sugars. You may omit this process when cooking lentils as they will not cause flatulence or indigestion.

It is preferable to soak beans overnight (in the refrigerator) as this will reduce the cooking time substantially. Undesirable legumes will float so skim the surface with a small strainer or slotted spoon to collect and discard them. Pour through a strainer and rinse before cooking. Replace water with fresh for cooking. You may change the water 2 or 3 times during soaking, to remove as much sugar as possible.

The cooking time required by legumes depends on how long they have been stored: the longer the storage time the greater the cooking time. Cooling time is also affected by the type of water used: i.e. with hard water, the softening process will take longer.

Once cooked, legumes can be kept in the refrigerator without deterioration for up to six to eight days, provided that they are stored in a different container than the one used for cooking. If you refrigerate them when still warm they are likely to become sour within days. Cooked legumes may be frozen in airtight containers for up to 3 months.

Chickpea and Sprout Salad

→ Soak the chickpeas in ½ cup of cold water overnight, place in the refrigerator. → The next day, drain then wash to remove all soaking water. → Bring 3 cups water to a boil in medium sized pan. → Add the bay leaf. → Next add the drained and washed chickpeas. → Bring back to a boil over high heat. Reduce heat to a simmer (low) and cook for only 10 minutes. → If it forms froth discard it with a slotted spoon.→ Cover the pan and continue cooking over medium heat for approximately 1 ½ to 2 hours. → The goal with the chickpeas is to attain an al dente texture so avoid over cooking. → To check, carefully remove one or two beans and verify that the center is still slightly firm. → Monitor the pan to insure that it doesn't run dry. If necessary **add more boiling hot water** (up to 2 or 3 times during cooking.) → Remove from heat at the end of the process. → Discard excess liquid. → Add salt in small amounts and mix well. → Let cool and serve.

Culinary note: Chickpeas are the only legume that requires the cooking water to be boiling prior to adding them to the pan. Water added during cooking process (if the pan starts to run dry) must also be hot / boiling. Other legumes may be placed in cold water to begin the cooking process. It is advised that water added during the cooking process is boiling to avoid cooling the pan and lengthening the cooking process.

Lentils with Vegetables

Bring 2 ½ cups of cold water to a boil in a medium pan. → Sort through the lentils discarding lentils that are not uniform. → Remove any stones. → Wash. → When water boils, add 1 bay leaf and washed and drained lentils. → Bring back to a boil, cover and cook over medium heat for about 20 minutes or until al dente. → If necessary, add **hot water** (½ cup) during cooking to prevent lentils from sticking together.

→ To know if lentils are al dente, carefully remove one or two lentils. → Check if they are cooked outside and very slightly uncooked inside. → Remove pot from the heat when done. → Set aside and continue with recipe instructions.

Culinary Note: It is important to monitor the cooking process, preventing the pan from going dry and also avoiding the addition of too much water. Ideally the lentils would be fully cooked and there would be no extra water left in the pan.

Culinary Note: It is important to monitor the cooking process, preventing water from evaporating or adding too much.

Medical note:
In some cases, legumes can cause flatulence because most contain some sugars that can cause digestive upset.
.

Hydrating sun-dried tomatoes

Used in recipes: Heart of Palm and Sun-dried Tomato Salad
Macaroni with Tofu and Mushrooms

Hydrate sun-dried tomatoes ... → Pour boiling water in a glass, ceramic or stainless steel bowl. → Place the sun-dried tomatoes in this water bath for a few minutes or until al dente. → Drain tomatoes in a colander. → Dry thoroughly. → Set aside. → Continue with the recipe instructions.

Washing (debittering) eggplant

Used in recipes: Hot vegetables
Eggplant, Pepper and Rosemary Salad
Eggplant a la Bolognese
Eggplants with Olives au Gratin (bubbly)

To eliminate the eggplant's bitter taste, it is necessary to follow the following procedure:

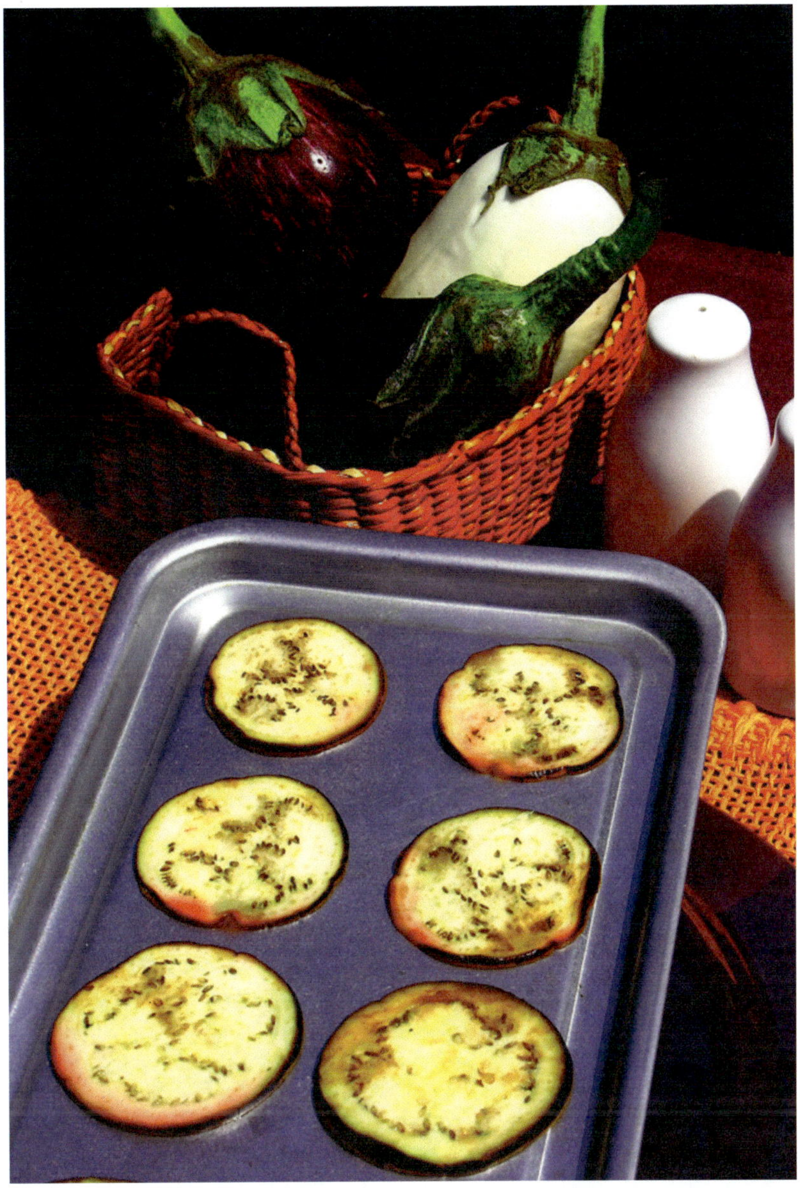

→ Wash eggplants and cut them as indicated in the recipe. → Arrange slices in layers on a plate or baking dish, one next to the other. → Spread or shake a small amount of salt on top the eggplant to remove bitterness. → Let stand for 20 minutes before cooking. → Rinse thoroughly under running water to remove salt. → Pat dry with paper towel and continue with the recipe instructions.

Culinary Note: If you need to do this procedure in advance of the final preparation of the recipe, coat the eggplant with lemon juice and then cover with salt to prevent discoloration.

Stuffing sweet potatoes

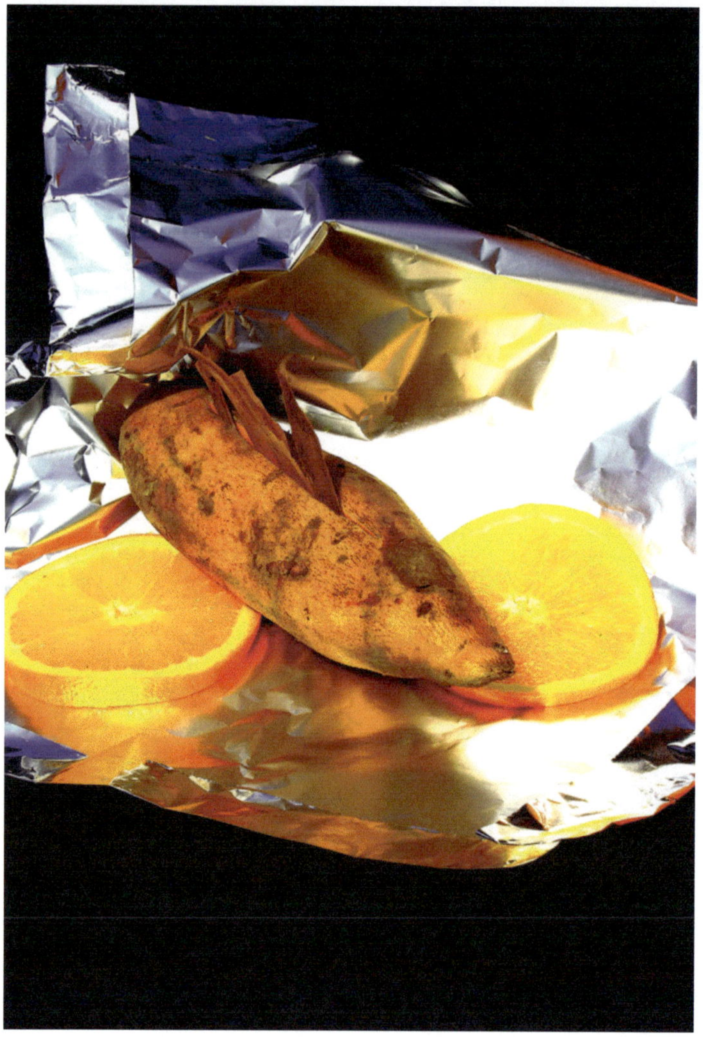

Used in recipe: Sweet Potato a L'Orange

→ Using a sharp knife make a longitudinal groove (½ inch - 1.23 cm. deep) in the sweet potato, deep enough to insert a cinnamon stick. → On the aluminum foil arrange the orange slices. Place the sweet potato on top and wrap tightly. → Continue with the recipe instructions.

Garlic oil

Used in recipe: Country-style Mashed Potatoes

With extra virgin olive oil: heat oven to 356 ° F or 180 ° C
With extra virgin avocado oil: heat stove to 491° F or 255° C

→ Place a nonstick pan on the burner set at medium heat. Add the amount of oil called for in the recipe. → Wait until oil is hot, but not smoking. → Add the garlic and sauté slowly for 3 minutes. → Cook the whole garlic evenly, first on one side and then on the other side. → Avoid unnecessary stirring allowing it to form a crust on the surface. → Remove pan from heat. → Discard the garlic. → Set aside the oil. → Continue with the recipe instructions.

Papillote (Baking Fish in a Foil Packet / Envelope)

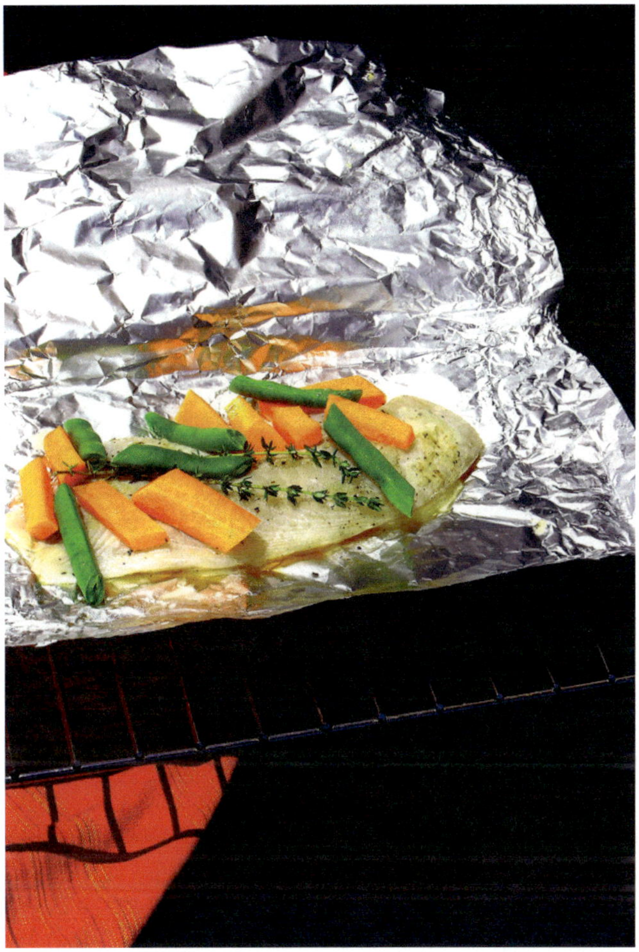

Used in recipe: Grilled or Baked Fish in Papillote

This technique is used for cooking food in its own juice, essentially the steam captured inside of the papillote (envelope). It is ideal for preserving nutrients, aromas and the flavors of food.

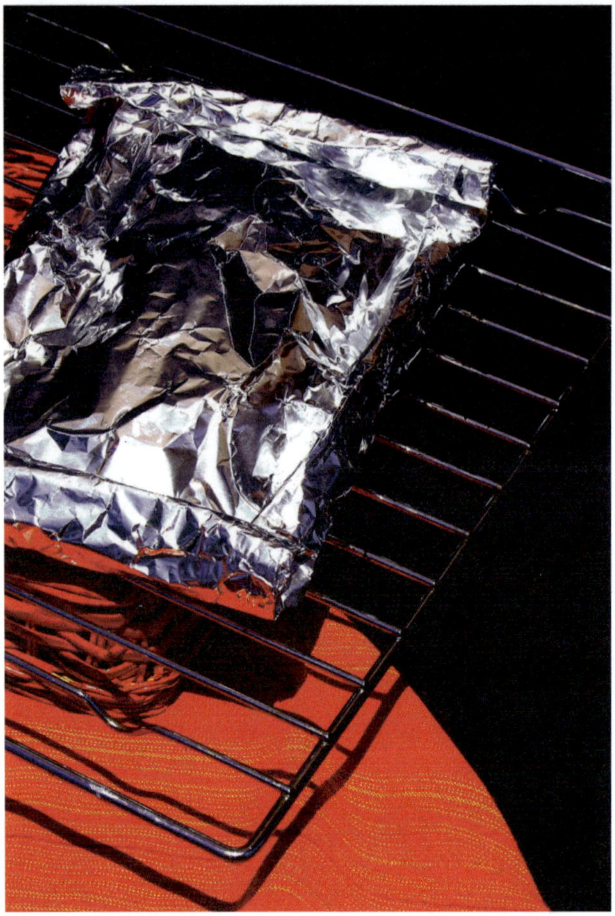

→ Cut a piece of foil that is twice the size of the piece of fish to be wrapped. → Place the filet at the end of the extended foil, leaving a small margin to fold. → Add the vegetables according to recipe instructions. → Cover with the other end of foil and close the three sides, forming the papillote. → Wrap the other filet using the same technique. → Continue with the recipe instructions.

Reducing liquids

Used in recipes: Basic Tomato Sauce
Orange, Cinnamon and Clove Gelatin

Reducing is the action of decreasing the amount of liquid in a preparation in order to intensify its flavor and make it thicker.

Basic Tomato Sauce

→ Continuously stir ingredients over minimum heat with a wooden spoon until half of the liquid evaporates and the sauce is slightly thickened. → Continue with the recipe instructions.

Orange, Cinnamon and Clove Gelatin

→ Continuously stir ingredients over minimum heat with a wooden spoon until a quarter of the liquid evaporates and slightly thickened. → Continue with the recipe instructions.

Important data:
Flavored or unflavored gelatin is an alternative method of hydration for patients who have difficulty swallowing liquids (dysphagia to liquids). It may also be used as a thickener for juices, shakes, etc., reducing the risk of causing the inhalation of liquids.

Searing rice

Used in recipe: Brown Rice with Vegetables

This technique is used so that the rice does not release starch during cooking process and the grains remain in whole and intact.

→ Heat oil in medium pan to 356 ° F or 180 ° C. → Add rice, previously washed and drained. → Stir constantly with a wooden spoon for 2 minutes or until rice becomes pearly or transparent. → Gradually add hot water, then add the raw vegetables. → Continue with the recipe instructions. →
Continue with the recipe instructions.

Roasting Peppers

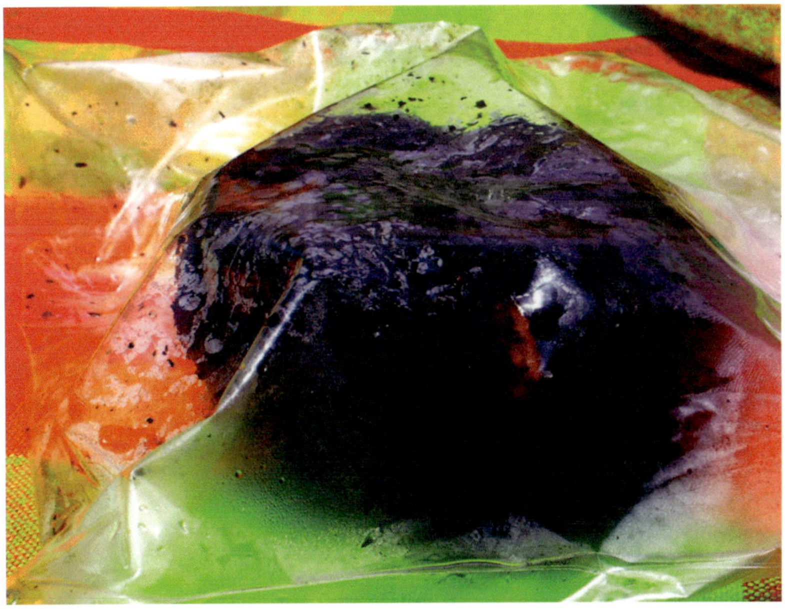

Used in recipes:	Olive, Pepper and Cottage Cheese Salad Eggplant, Pepper and Rosemary salad Baby Spinach Salad

The skin of the pepper will be easily removed using this method.

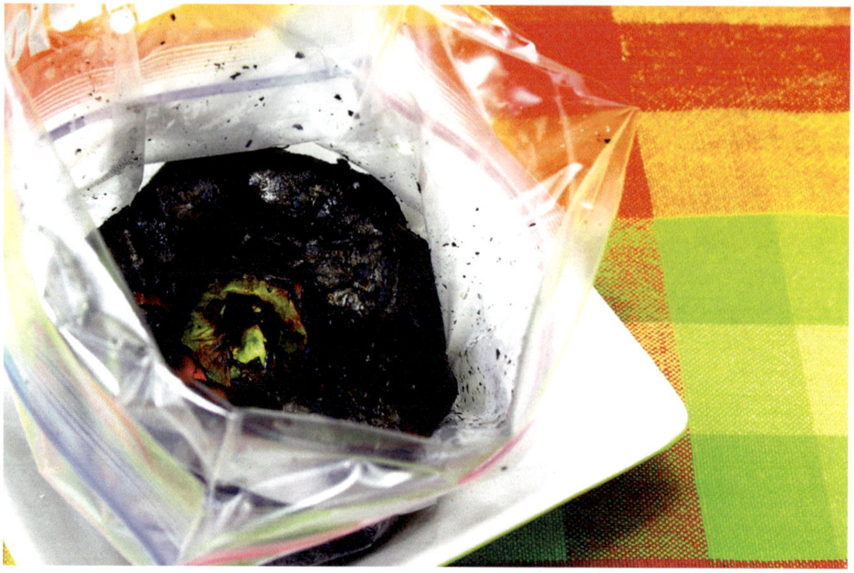

Vapors allow to separate pepper skin easily.

This roasting peppers technique can be done on a gas stove or grill, until skin of peppers is completely burned.

On the gas stove:

→ Select the color pepper you prefer and wash it. → Securely insert a long handled fork to hold and rotate the pepper during roasting. → Hold the pepper over the gas flame and burn all the skin surface evenly. You might wish to place a plate nearby to deposit the roasted pepper when done or in the event that it comes off the fork.→ Place the hot and blackened pepper into a plastic bag. → Close tightly until the pepper is cool. → Rub the pepper with your hands inside the bag to peel skin. → Remove from bag and wipe with a paper towel to completely eliminate the burnt skin. → Do not wash the pepper with water as it will cause it to lose its natural oils.

On the grill:

→ Select the color pepper you prefer and wash it. → Grab the pepper with grill tongs and place on the preheated and hot grill. Turn and blacken on all sides, taking approximately 10 minutes. → Place the hot and totally blackened pepper into a plastic bag. → Close tightly until the pepper is cool. → Rub the pepper with your hands inside the bag to peel the skin. → Remove from bag and wipe with a paper towel to completely eliminate the burnt skin. → Do not wash the pepper with water as it will cause it to lose its natural oils.

Important note for the patient:
It is not advisable to consume the burnt skin from peppers.

Culinary note: the smoky flavor of the roasted pepper is delicious. We recommend cutting them into pieces, dress with a small amount of olive oil and season with moderation. They can be served at room temperature in salads or as an accompaniment to fish and poultry.

Toasting sesame seeds

Used in recipe: Assorted Fruits

→ Heat a non-stick frying pan to minimum heat and add the sesame seeds. → Stir constantly until slightly browned. → Allow to cool and use. → They can be kept refrigerated in an airtight container up to 30 days.

Cooking with oils

Medical and culinary recommendation: Do not use these cooking methods if you want to lose weight. When frying, sautéing or browning foods, they are impregnated with oil and increase caloric value. However, there are some recipes in which this procedure is essential.

Heating oils at lower temperature conditions the avocado and extra virgin olive oil show no substantial change in its structure and conserve their original properties better than other healthy oils. If overheated, oils reach what is called the smoke point which indicates the breakdown of the fat which is an unhealthy outcome.

Extra virgin olive oil:	smoke point: 356° F or 180° C
Extra virgin avocado oil:	smoke point: 491° F or 255° C

If the oil is not hot enough when the food is added it becomes impregnated with excessive oil, is indigestible and will not be crisp. The immersion in oil at the proper temperature creates a thin outer crust, which stops further oil penetration. It also helps to retain the natural moisture inside of the food.

On the contrary, if the oil is too hot (beyond the smoke point), it vaporizes and smokes, thereby altering its properties and becoming harmful to health.

To measure the temperature of the oil, we suggest a "liquid food thermometer" though you will eventually be able to gauge the temperature without a thermometer.

Foods should be cooked dry. It is also convenient to use small pieces so that temperature quickly reaches the center of the portion. Avoid a prolonged frying.

Browning

Used in recipes: Eggplant a la Bolognese
Neapolitan-Style Mushrooms
Broccoli Crêpe
Lentils with Vegetables
Macaroni with Tofu and Mushrooms
Potatoes with Parsley
Grilled Fish
Neapolitan-style Baked Chicken
Chicken Sauté with Vegetables
Basic Tomato Sauce
Spaghetti with Vegetables and Olives
Zucchini au Gratin with Mushrooms

Browning is the cooking process through which foods obtain a characteristic "golden" color.

The technique consists on exposing for a few minutes the outer layer of food to a source of intense heat, so it stays crisp and golden also retains its moisture content. The fried food color is golden yellow to coppery brown.

For browning:

With extra virgin olive oil: heat oil to 356 ° F or 180 ° C
With extra virgin avocado oil: heat oil to 491 ° F or 255 ° C

→ Place a non-stick frying pan on the stovetop heat and add the amount of oil called for in the recipe. → Wait for the oil heat. → Add piece(s) to the pan using tongs or a long handled fork. → In some recipes it will be necessary to occasionally stir or turn the ingredients or pieces so it browns evenly. → Remove ingredients from frying pan and allow to rest on several layers of paper towel which will absorb excess fat.

Frying

Used in recipes: Neapolitan-Style Mushrooms
Broccoli Crêpe
Chicken or Turkey Burger
Pork Loin with Sage
Breaded Chicken or Turkey Cutlets (Milanese)
Vegetable Omelet
Potatoes with Parsley

Frying is cooking food by submerging it in oil or other fat, at a given temperature until fully cooked. The color of frying is usually light brown to dark brown.

For frying:

With extra virgin olive oil: heat oil to 356 ° F or 180 ° C
With extra virgin avocado oil: heat oil to 491 ° F or 255 ° C

→ Place a non-stick frying pan on the stovetop and add the amount of oil called for in the recipe. → Wait for the oil heat fully. → Place the pieces in the frying pan with tongs or a long handled fork. → Cook evenly, first on one side and then on the other. → Avoid unnecessarily moving so that a crust will form on the surface. → Remove from the frying pan and place on several layers of paper towel to absorb excess fat.

Sautéing

Used in recipes: Spinach and Mushroom Salad in Soy Sauce
Chickpea and Sprout Salad
Hot Vegetables
Potatoes with Parsley
Neapolitan Style Baked Chicken
Chicken Sauté with Vegetables
Basic Tomato Sauce
Tomato and Thyme Soup
Spinach and Mushroom Soufflé

Sautéing is a fast paced method of cooking which utilizes a small amount of oil in a frying pan or saucepan. The outside is lightly browned and inside is lightly cooked. In general, sautéing is used for low-volume parts, stirring constantly to avoid cooking them completely. Ingredients are generally cut into pieces or thinly sliced. The color of sautéed food is pale yellow.

For sautéing:

With extra virgin olive oil:	heat oil to 356 ° F or 180 ° C
With avocado extra virgin oil:	heat oil to 491 ° F or 255 ° C

→ Place a non-stick frying pan on the stove top and add the amount of oil called for in the recipe. → Wait for the oil to heat. → Arrange piece(s) with tongs or a long handled fork. → Brown slightly on the outside and remove from pan. → Place on several layers of paper towels which will remove excess oil. Allow to rest.

Important tips when using oils

It is not recommended to mix new and old oil, nor the avocado with olive oil or other seed oils or fats. The oils have different smoke points and may produce irritating and potentially toxic substances when heated together.

Used oil should be discarded in closed plastic bags in the trash. This not only pollutes the water, it also damages pipes.

In the event of a fire in the kitchen caused by overheated cooking oils, do not use water to extinguish it as it may explode. Keep a fire extinguisher handy in the kitchen just to be safe.

Oven cooking technique

Gratinéing (Au Gratin, Bubbly)

Used in recipes: Eggplant a la Bolognese
Eggplants with Olives au Gratin (bubbly)
Neapolitan-style Baked Chicken
Zucchini with Mushrooms au Gratin

Gratinéing (Au gratin, Bubbly) is a cooking technique applied to foods that are cooked in oven. The technique consists in exposing the outer layer of the preparation to an intense source of heat, so it becomes crispy and golden. The purpose of gratinéing is to develop a thin covering that protects and maintains the aroma of cooked ingredients. Generally, the gratin is applied in the recipes which at the end were sprinkled with cheese bread crumbs or some other ingredient that can get a golden color.

In the recipes of this book, gratin is the final finishing given to some foods that, generally, have been previously baked.

→ Keep preparation in hot oven (390 ° F or 200 ° C), i.e. without removing from the oven when it is cooked. → Wait until it forms a golden crust on the surface. → Remove carefully and bring to the table. → Serve immediately to keep its crispy texture.

Culinary Note: we recommended monitoring the process, since oven temperatures can vary according to model.

Oven temperatures used in the recipes

Low	approximately	250° F	120° C
Medium low	approximately	320° F	160° C
Medium	approximately	350° F	180° C
Medium High	approximately	390° F	200° C
High	approximately	450° F	230° C

Measures and equivalences used in the recipes

Simple measures and equivalents used in the recipes in this book

1 teaspoon	5 milliliters	
1 tablespoon	3 teaspoons	
1 tablespoon	15 milliliters	1/2 fluid ounce
2 tablespoons	30 milliliters	1 fluid ounce
1 cup	16 tablespoons	
1 cup	240 milliliters	8 fluid ounces

Additional Recommendations

A healthy bar-b-que

The consumption of meat cooked on high heat resulting in the blackening of the outside (carbonization) is associated with the development of gastrointestinal cancer.

Before using the bar-b-que

Searing the meat is recommended prior to placing it on the grill. This reduces the exposure to the direct heat of the bar-b-que and seals in the juices. Another way of grilling is to utilize a grill made of a flat, metal surface. One can also wrap the sealed meat in aluminum foil and place it on the grill.

Searing food: is a procedure that is often used when the pieces are large and thick (roast pork, thick chicken breasts, fish fillets or meat).

With extra virgin olive oil:	heat to 356 ° F or 180 ° C
With avocado extra virgin oil:	heat to 491 ° F or 255 ° C

→ Place a non-stick frying pan or skillet on the burner and add 1 tablespoon of oil. → Wait for the oil to heat. → Carefully place the pieces of meat, fish or poultry in the frying pan using tongs or a longhandled fork. → Sear by frying quickly. → When a thin, brown crust has formed, carefully turn it over and sear it on the other side. → Repeat browning all sides. → Remove the seared pieces from pan and move to the grill to complete the cooking process.

Peeling raw tomatoes

→ Wash tomatoes well. → With a sharp knife cut a shallow X in the skin. Locate the cut on the side opposite to the stem, the bottom or widest part of the tomato. → Drop in a bowl of hot water for 2 minutes. → Remove with a slotted spoon and then submerge in a bowl with ice water for 30 seconds. → Remove from cold water bath and peel. → Tomato skin opens at the cross cut and can be easily removed with your fingers. → If you want to discard the seeds, cut tomato in half and remove with a spoon.

HERBS, SPICES AND CONDIMENTS

Uses as a dietary supplement for weight loss

The use of spices and aromatic herbs in the diet allow the development of low-salt dishes that are healthier and tastier.

Mediterranean cuisine in general prefers to keep the original food's taste and aroma. However, we recommend using some of these species and herbs to enhance the food flavors.

Some recommendations:
Fresh herbs are kept in good condition for a week or two in a closed plastic container with water in the refrigerator. But dried herbs, which have a more intense flavor, can be stored for several months at room temperature.

During food preparation it is preferable to use small amounts, especially if using dried herbs. To combine them properly it is necessary to know some of their characteristics.

From the culinary point of view we distinguish the following herbs, spices and condiments that we can use.

AROMATIC HERBS

BASIL: Use leaves, dried or frozen. It is the ideal complement to dishes made with tomatoes, eggs and cheese.

SAFFRON: Use the dried stigmas of the plant, which are sold in both strands and powder. This spice is one of the most expensive and is often used to give it a characteristic taste to the rice, poultry, seafood and fish.

CUMIN: Use the fruits of the plant, which look alike seeds. It is used as a seasoning for all meats, cheeses and vegetables.

CORIANDER / cilantro: Use the leaves, the seeds and the root, in some places. It is used fresh and dried to flavor the fish.

DILL: Use the leaves and fruits that combine well with fish, poultry, vegetables and boiled potatoes.

FENNEL: Use the whole plant, bulbs, leaves and seeds. It is used to flavor salads, fish, poultry, vegetables, soups and sauces.

BAY LEAVE: Use fresh or dried leaves in preparing tomato sauces and meat dishes. Leaves are removed before serving.

MARJORAM: The leaves used are fresh or dried, whole or powdered. It is confused with oregano because of its appearance but is lighter, with a more delicate flavor. Goes well with poultry, salads, vegetables and eggs.

OREGANO: Use fresh or dried leaves, which give a special flavor to pasta, pizza, preparations made from tomatoes and cheese. It also accentuates the flavor of baked chicken.

PARSLEY: Use leaves and stems; widely used, preferably consumed fresh. Highlights soups, sautéed vegetables flavors etc.

ROSEMARY: Use leaves, fresh or dried. It has an intense flavor and is an excellent condiment for grilled poultry and casseroles with tomato.

SAGE: Leaves are used fresh or dry and should not be mixed with other herbs. It is used to flavor poultry and sauces.

THYME: Use fresh or dried leaves, which go well with eggs, poultry, seafood, pasta and the preparation of tomato sauces.

GREEN TEA: Leaves are pressed and crushed in the sun. One of the most beneficial effects of green tea is that it inhibits the oxidation of LDL (good blood fat) in the arteries, which can counteract the formation of atherosclerosis. It can be taken hot or cold, and is a healthy alternative to sodas. Green tea contains a high amount of caffeine; we recommend a moderate intake to avoid insomnia. Certain substances in green tea can cause gastritis if you drink it too concentrated.

SPECIES:

CINNAMON: It is the dried bark of the cinnamon tree and is used in sticks or powder to flavor desserts, fresh fruit, punch, hot drinks and some desserts.

CLOVES: Are dried flower buds (whole or grounded) of some shrubs or trees species. It is recommended to use moderately in desserts that include fruit and some sauces.

MUSTARD: Ground seeds are used to prepare the paste-like condiment known as mustard. It is used to flavor chicken and salads.

NUTMEG: The seeds of the plant are used dry and grated in the preparation of hot drinks, fruit compotes and sauces.

BLACK PEPPER: Immature berries, sun-dried, granulated or powdered are used in most meals.

VANILLA: It is a flavoring substance elaborated from the seed pods. It is used in all kinds of desserts, hot and cold drinks.

ACIDIC CONDIMENTS & SPICES:

VINEGAR: Derives from the activity of the bacteria acetyl *Mycoderma* that performs the chemical reaction converting by fermentation the ethyl alcohol (wine) to acetic acid (vinegar). To achieve this transformation, there most be appropriate conditions of acidity, alcohol and nutrient concentration.

BALSAMIC VINEGAR or Balsamic Aceto: The best known aceto is the Balsamic Aceto di Modena, which is a type of vinegar from the Italian region of Emilia-Romagna. Especially made in the city which gives its name: Modena.

The process to prepare the balsamic vinegar starts when boiling grape juice until it becomes a thick intensely flavored **sugary** syrup, with a dark and slightly sweet flavor. It is generally used as a substitute in foods containing wine, because it provides a similar flavor.

APPLE VINEGAR: It has been used for years because of its great diuretic effect. It is rich in potassium and has a purifying effect.

RICE VINEGAR OR MIRIN (gastronomy): It is a mild vinegar produced by fermentation of rice. Widely used in Japanese cuisine, has a subtle flavor and is lighter than other vinegars, but it could retain fluids.

ALLIACEAE-BASED SEASONINGS:

GARLIC: Cooked bulbs have a delicate taste and are used in the preparation of many foods.

ONION: Use raw or cooked in salads, pasta, stews and all types of birds and fish.

HOT CONDIMENTS & SPICES:

HOT PEPPER yellow or special (*Capsicum chinense*): It is native from Peru and is one of the most widely used spices in Peruvian cuisine. It is a large spicy fruit, usually red, although there are other colors. It is used whole or grounded as a condiment.

Red hot peppers are rich in vitamins A and C and contain potassium, magnesium and iron. Green or yellow peppers have fewer vitamins than red.

Hot pepper favors the opening of taste buds, giving rise to segregation of saliva and gastric juices that stimulate the appetite.

CHILE:
It is a spicy fruit par excellence, associated to the Mexican culture, being an essential food in their gastronomy. It has been subject of scientific studies that have shown its cleansing properties.

Originally from Mexico, where it is called chilli. It comprises more than 150 varieties, being the prototype species *Capsicum annuum*. Its greatest use is done in Aztec lands, although it has a large market in Central America, Southeast Asia (Korea, India, Pakistan and Thailand), United States and Eastern Europe.

As a matter of information, it is important to mention that in places, like in the U.S., the grown peppers are not spicy, and are commonly known as Bell Pepper. They are mainly used in salads and sometimes are used stuffed with meat and cheese.

CAYENNE PEPPER:
Cayenne Pepper comes from a shrub whose fruits are hot or chili peppers, which are subsequently dried to grind them. The chili powder extracted by grinding is known as cayenne pepper (named after the city of Cayenne, French Guiana).

Tender chiles or peppers are yellow, and become red as they mature. Once dry, they take on a maroon or dark red color. Another variety is the tabasco, from which tabasco sauce is made.

CURRY:
The name "curry" comes from India and means stew. The “mixture of curry” often includes the following species: red pepper, basil, caraway (similar to fennel), cardamom, turmeric, fenugreek (herb from India), saffron, cinnamon, dried onion, celery, cilantro, cumin, ginger, mustard, nutmeg, cayenne pepper, black pepper and tamarind. The curry recipe varies according to each region and its color depends on the mixture ingredients.

PRACTICAL-MEDICAL GUIDE FOR MENUS AND RECIPES
Medical Recommendations to vary the menu ingredients

- Diabetes
- Vascular Disease
- Heart disease
- Celiac disease
- Gout (uric acid)
- Hypertension
- Hyperlipidemia
- Kidney stones (calcium oxalate and/or sodium urate)
- *Rheumatic Disease*

Use the recipes of this book varying the amount and/or ingredients as described below:

First Courses and Appetizers

NATURAL-STYLE TUNA

Medical note: wash tuna with fresh water to remove excess salt.

NEAPOLITAN-STYLE MUSHROOMS

Diabetics: halve or quarter the amount of onion (high sugar content) and remove the cooking water (sodium).

Gouties: dialyze* mushrooms and remove the cooking water (high purines and sodium content).

Hypertensives: dialyze* mushrooms and remove the cooking water (high sodium content).

BROCCOLI CRÊPE

Cardiacs: dialyze* 2 times the broccoli (mineral content).

Hyperlipemics: replace one of the yolks with an egg white.

Kidney Stones: reduce the amount of broccoli (oxalate) or replace it with cauliflower or zucchini.

- Cauliflower Crêpe

Hyperlipemics: replace one of the yolks with an egg white.

Medical note: cauliflower can produce gases; we recommend antiflatulents before eating it.

- Pepper Crêpe

Hyperlipemics: replace one of the yolks with an egg white.

- Green Bean Crêpe

Hyperlipemics: replace one of the yolks with an egg white.

VEGETABLE OMELET

Diabetics: replace green peas and carrots with green beans (high sugar content).
Gouties: replace green peas with green beans (purines content).
Hyperlipemics: replace one of the yolks with an egg white.
Kidney stones: halve the amount of carrots (oxalate content).

- Mushrooms Omelet

Gouties: dialyze* mushrooms and remove the cooking water (high purines and sodium content).
Hypertensives: dialyze* mushrooms and remove the cooking water (high sodium content).
Hyperlipemics: replace one of the yolks with an egg white.

- Turkey ham Omelet

Gouties: dialyze* mushrooms and remove the cooking water (high purines and sodium content). Do not increase the amount of turkey ham.
Hyperlipemics: replace one of the yolks with an egg white.

- Cheese Omelet

Hyperlipemics: replace one of the yolks with an egg white

VEGETABLES IN COLD OREGANO SAUCE

Diabetics: replace corn and carrots (high sugar content) with blanched zucchini and cauliflower.
Kidney stones: halve the amount of carrots (oxalate content) and replace the tomatoes and zucchini with broccoli and cauliflower.

Medical note: To prevent digestive disorders, use skinned and seeded tomatoes.

POKER OF VEGETABLES À LA CRÈME

Diabetes: halve the amount of beetroot (high sugar content).
Cardiacs: halve the amount of beetroot (high sugar content contributes to cardiac risk.)
Hypertensives: halve the amount of beetroot (high sugar content contributes to cardiovascular risk.)
Kidney Stones: avoid this combination of vegetables (oxalate content).

Medical note: beetroot can promote fluid retention due to its high content of sugar and salts. Not recommended for patients who want to lose weight.

SPINACH AND MUSHROOMS SOUFFLÉ

Vascular Disease: dialyze* 3 times spinach (mineral content).
Cardiacs: dialyze* 3 times spinach (mineral content).
Gouties: avoid spinach and mushrooms (purine content).
Hypertensives: dialyze* mushrooms and remove the cooking water (sodium content).
Kidney Stones: replace spinach (oxalate content) with cauliflower.
Medical note: unsalted butter contains 19 calories per 1/2 tsp; salt butter contains 18.5 calories. This factor is because unsalted butter concentrates proteins and nutrients.

Sides

BROWN RICE WITH VEGETABLES

Diabetics: replace green peas and carrots (high sugar content) with ¼ cup red pepper and ¼ cup green peppers, skinned, cut into squares.
Gouties: replace green peas and carrots (high concentration of purines) with ¼ cup red pepper and ¼ cup green peppers, skinned, cut into squares.
Kidney stones: halve the amount of green peas and carrots (oxalate content).

HOT VEGETABLES

Diabetics: exclude butter.
Cardiacs: exclude butter.
Gouties: dialyze* 3 times the vegetables and mushrooms (high concentration of purine).
Hypertensives: exclude butter.
Hyperlipemics: exclude butter.
Kidney Stones: avoid this combination of vegetables (oxalate content).
Rheumatics: exclude butter.
Medical note: cauliflower can produce gases; we recommend antiflatulents before eating it.

BAKED OR GRILLED POTATO

Diabetics: halve or quarter the amount of potatoes (high sugar content).
Cardiacs: halve or quarter the amount of potatoes (sugar contributes to cardiovascular risk.)
Hypertensives: halve or quarter the amount of potatoes (sugar contributes to cardiovascular risk, can increase cardiac activity and raise blood pressure).
Hyperlipemics: halve or quarter the amount of potatoes because the consumption of carbohydrates increases triglycerides.
Kidney stones: halve or quarter the amount of potatoes (oxalate content).

SMALL POTATOES WITH PARSLEY

Diabetics: halve or quarter the amount of potatoes (high sugar content).
Cardiacs: halve or quarter the amount of potatoes (high sugar content) because it can increase cardiac activity.
Hypertensives: halve or quarter the amount of potatoes (high sugar content) because it can increase cardiac activity and raise blood pressure.
Hyperlipemics: exclude the butter (increases LDL "bad" cholesterol) and halve or quarter the amount of potatoes because it can increase triglycerides.
Kidney stones: halve or quarter the amount of potatoes (high oxalate content).

SMALL BAKED POTATOES WITH EXTRA VIRGIN OLIVE OIL

Diabetics: halve or quarter the amount of potatoes (high sugar content).

Cardiacs: halve or quarter the amount of potatoes (high sugar content) because it can increase cardiac activity.

Hypertensives: halve or quarter the amount of potatoes (high sugar content) because it can increase cardiac activity and raise blood pressure.

Hyperlipemics: halve or quarter the amount of potatoes because it can increase triglycerides.

Kidney stones: halve or quarter the amount of potatoes (oxalate content).

SPINACH PURÉE

Diabetics: halve the amount of potatoes (high sugar content).

Vascular Disease: dialyze* 3 times spinach (mineral content).

Gouties: not recommended the spinach (purine content).

Hypertensives: the fiber present in the spinach helps, as it slows the absorption of the potato's sugar.

Hyperlipemics: dialyze* 3 times spinach (mineral content).

Kidney stones: not recommended the consumption of spinach (purines).

COUNTRY-STYLE MASHED POTATOES

Diabetics: halve or quarter the amount of potatoes (high sugar content).

Cardiacs: halve or quarter the amount of potatoes (high sugar content) because it can increase cardiac activity.

Hypertensives: halve or quarter the amount of potatoes (high sugar content) because it can increase cardiac activity and raise blood pressure.

Hyperlipemics: exclude the butter (increases LDL "bad" cholesterol) and halve or quarter the amount of potatoes because it can increase triglycerides.

Kidney stones: halve or quarter the amount of potatoes and garlic (oxalate content).

GLAZED CARROTS

Diabetics: not recommended because of high sugar content in carrots and raisins.

Cardiacs: not recommended because high sugar content in carrots and raisins can increase cardiac activity and raise blood pressure.

Hypertensives: not recommended because high sugar content in carrots and raisins can increase cardiac activity and raise blood pressure.

Hyperlipemics: exclude butter (cholesterol).

Kidney stones: halve or quarter the amount of carrot and cinnamon (oxalates).

Medical note: despite the low caloric value of the recipe, the artificial sweetener splenda retains fluids. If you do not need to lose weight, you can replace the sweetener by 1/3 cup of brown sugar.

Salads

CABBAGE, CARROT AND RAISIN CHINESE SALAD

Diabetics: not recommended because of high sugar content in carrots and raisins.

Cardiacs: exclude raisins (high sugar content) because they may increase cardiac activity.

Hypertensives: exclude raisins (high sugar content) because they may increase cardiac activity and raise blood pressure.

Kidney Stones: decrease the amount of carrots (oxalate content).

***Medical note*:** If you do not need to lose weight, you can substitute ¼ teaspoon of splenda per ¼ tsp of brown sugar.

OLIVE, PEPPER AND COTTAGE CHEESE SALAD

Diabetes: eat onion with caution because its sugar content can cause hyperglycaemia.

Hypertensives: do not accompany this recipe with more protein.

Kidney stones: halve the amount of lettuce and onions (oxalate content).

EGGPLANT, PEPPER AND ROSEMARY SALAD

Kidney stones: not recommended because of oxalate content in vegetables.

ASPARAGUS AND BROCCOLI SALAD

Diabetics: the corn can be included because the ingredients of the recipe have enough fiber to slow the increase in blood sugar.

Gouties: replace asparagus (purines content) with zucchini.

BABY SPINACH SALAD

Gouties: spinach not recommended (purines content).

Kidney stones: spinach not recommended (oxalate content).

SPINACH AND MUSHROOMS SALAD IN SOY SAUCE

Vascular disease: exclude mushrooms, soy sauce and salt excess.

Cardiacs: exclude mushrooms, soy sauce and salt excess.

Gouties: spinach not recommended (purines).

Hypertensives: exclude mushrooms, soy sauce and salt excess.

Kidney stones: spinach not recommended (oxalate content).

CHICKPEA AND SPROUT SALAD

Diabetics: replace green peas and carrots (mineral content) with zucchini and green beans.

Gouties: replace the chickpeas (purines) with rice.

Kidney stones: replace the chickpeas (oxalate content) with rice.

HEART OF PALM AND SUN-DRIED TOMATO SALAD

Diabetics: exclude croutons (carbohydrates).

Celiac: exclude croutons (carbohydrates).

Gouties: not recommended because of purines in hart of palm.

Hypertensives: not recommended because dehydrated tomatoes have high sugar content and spinach and palms contain mineral.

Kidney stones: not recommended because of oxalate content in the mix of vegetables.

AVOCADO, LETTUCE AND TOMATO SALAD

Diabetics: exclude the corn (high sugar content).

Cardiacs: not recommended because the avocado is high in calories and corn has a high sugar concentration that can increase cardiac activity.

Hypertensives: not recommended because the avocado is high in calories and corn has a high sugar concentration that can increase cardiac activity and raise blood pressure.

CHICKEN, ASPARAGUS AND APPLE SALAD

Gouties: exclude asparagus (purines content).

Medical note: we recommend peeling the apples, since the skin contains pectin which is not soluble; it takes time to be digested and can cause gas. The red skin contains more calories than the green skin. Consume only the tips of the asparagus because the fibrous part of the plant can hinder digestion.

CHERRY TOMATO AND NUT SALAD

MIXED GREEN VEGETABLE, FETA CHEESE AND PECAN SALAD

Diabetics: exclude croutons (carbohydrates).

Celiac: exclude croutons (carbohydrates).

Hyperlipemics: exclude croutons because bread raises triglycerides.

Kidney stones: exclude pecans (oxalate content).

Soups and Creams

CHICKEN BREAST BROTH

Diabetics: exclude noodles (high carbohydrate content).

Celiac: use gluten-free noodles.

Kidney stones: exclude celery (oxalate content).

CREAM OF MUSHROOMS SOUP

Gouties: not recommended because mushrooms contain a considerable amount of purines.

CREAM OF MIXED VEGETABLE SOUP

Gouties: green peas not recommended (purines).

Kidney stones: green peas not recommended (oxalate content).

TOMATO AND THYME SOUP

Kidney stones: exclude celery (oxalate content).

Sandwiches

CAPRESE SANDWICH

Diabetics: exclude bread; eat mozzarella and tomato with basil and olive oil.
Celiac: use gluten-free bread.

OLIVE AND HARD-BOILED EGG SANDWICH

Diabetics: exclude bread; eat olives and egg with mustard and mayonnaise.
Celiac: use gluten-free bread.

TUNA SANDWICH

Diabetics: exclude bread; eat tuna and lettuce with mayonnaise and mustard.
Celiac: use gluten-free bread.

***Medical note*:** wash the contents of the tuna can with three jets of hot water to remove all salt.

EGG AND CHIVE OR CIBOULETTES SANDWICH

Diabetics: exclude bread; eat egg and chives with mayonnaise and mustard.
Celiac: use gluten-free bread.

TURKEY OR HAM SANDWICH

Diabetics: exclude bread; eat turkey or ham with mustard.
Celiac: use gluten-free bread.
Gouties: do not increase the amount of turkey ham.

CHICKEN SANDWICH

Diabetics: exclude bread; eat the chicken with mayonnaise and celery.
Celiac: use gluten-free bread.
Kidney stones: do not increase the amount of celery.

SALMON SANDWICH

Diabetics: exclude bread; eat salmon and ricotta cheese with capers and olive oil.
Celiac: use gluten-free bread.
Hypertensives: exclude salt and pepper.

***Medical note*:** salmon and capers packed contain significant amounts of salt. Wash twice with cold water.

TRICOLOR SANDWICH

Diabetics: exclude bread; eat the tomato and avocado with mayonnaise.
Celiac: use gluten-free bread.

HOT OR COLD HAM AND CHEESE SANDWICH

Diabetics: exclude bread; eat mozzarella cheese and ham.
Celiac: use gluten-free bread.
Gouties: do not increase the amount of ham.

Main Courses

BOLOGNESE-STYLE EGGPLANT

Kidney stones: not recommended because of high oxalate content in eggplant.

CHICKEN OR TURKEY BURGER

Celiac: use gluten-free bread.
Gouties: do not increase the amount of turkey ham.

BREADED CHICKEN OR TURKEY CUTLETS (MILANESE)

Celiac: use gluten-free crackers.
Kidney stones: do not increase the amount of protein.

CURRY CHICKEN WITH MINT

BAKED CHICKEN WITH ROSEMARY

NEAPOLITAN-STYLE BAKED CHICKEN

Gouties: not recommended because of purines content in the combination of these vegetables.
Kidney stones: spinach not recommended (oxalate content).

CHICKEN SAUTÉ WITH VEGETABLES

Cardiacs: exclude salt and soy sauce.
Kidney Stones: exclude soybean (oxalate content).

Medical note**:** the use of soy sauce should be dosed because of its salt concentration. Salt excess in this recipe is offset by the properties of apple cider vinegar, which is a natural diuretic.

GRILLED OR BAKED FISH EN PAPILLOTE

Gouties: do not to increase the amount of protein.

GRIDDLED FISH

Gouties: do not to increase the amount of protein.
Kidney stones: quarter the amount of garlic (oxalate content).

MEDITERRANEAN SALMON

Cardiacs: exclude capers and salt.
Kidney stones: do not increase the amount of protein.

***Medical note*:** In general, we recommend to wash the capers and not to add salt to the recipe.

EGGPLANT WITH OLIVES AU GRATIN

Gouties: replace the cheeses with half grilled chicken breast.
Kidney stones: eggplant not recommended (oxalate content).

PORK LOIN WITH SAGE

Cardiacs: exclude butter.
Gouties: do not increase the amount of pork.
Hyperlipemics: exclude butter.

LENTILS WITH VEGETABLES

Gouties: lentils not recommended because of its purines content.

***Medical note*:** not recommendable for patients with gastritis because it can make difficult the digestion of beans. Do not to add another class of proteins to the recipe. After eating the soup, it is suggested to have a cup of anise to facilitate digestion. The protein from beans eaten with rice, greens, lemon and foods with high vitamin B12, forms haemoglobin.

MACARONI WITH TOFU AND MUSHROOMS

Diabetics: not recommended because flour contains large amounts of sugar.
Cardiacs: exclude butter.
Celiac: use gluten-free pasta.
Gouties: not recommended because of mushrooms and soy purine content.
Hypertensives: not recommended because of salt content in mushrooms and noodles.
Kidney stones: not recommended because of oxalate content in tofu.

SPAGHETTI WITH VEGETABLES AND OLIVES

Diabetics: not recommended because flour contains large amounts of sugar.
Cardiacs: halve the portion because of salts content in the recipe ingredients.
Celiac: replace with gluten-free pasta.
Hypertensives: exclude salt and soybeans.
Kidney stones: exclude soy.

ZUCCHINI AU GRATIN WITH MUSHROOMS

Gouties: not recommended because of purine content in mushrooms.

Salad Dressings and Sauces*

PEPPER OIL

LEMON DRESSING

Diabetics: exclude sugar and use splenda because it can produce moderate fluid retention.
Vascular desease: exclude soy.
Cardiacs: exclude soy.
Gouties: exclude soy.
Hypertensives: exclude soy.
Kidney stones: exclude soy.

HOMEMADE MAYONNAISE

***Medical note*:** Because of its high-calorie content, dilute suggested portion with water.

HOMEMADE MAYONNAISE WITH CURRY

***Medical note*:** Because of its high-caloric content, dilute suggested portion with water.

BASIC TOMATO SAUCE

***Medical note*:** the acidity of tomato is neutralized by the olive or avocado oil, so that patients with gastritis can consume it.

SWEET AND SOUR VINAIGRETTE

Diabetics: exclude the honey.

Desserts and Drinks

SWEET POTATO A L'ORANGE

Diabetics: exclude port and sugar.
Hyperlipemics: exclude butter.

ASSORTED FRUITS WITH YOGURT, HONEY AND SESAME

Diabetics: do not eat watermelon, grapes or mango because of its high sugar content.
Kidney Stones: replace papaya strawberries, and mandarin with peaches, blackberries and raspberries ½ pineapple and banana. Exclude grapes.

Suggested accompaniments

Diabetics: exclude honey and prunes (high sugar content).
Kidney Stones: exclude sesame (oxalate content).

Medical note: consume lemonade prepared with a lemon juice diluted in a glass of water, up to 2 times a day.

ORANGE, CINNAMON AND CLOVE GELATIN

Diabetics: Replace the orange with blended peach.
Kidney Stones: Replace the orange with blended peach.

STRAWBERRY FRAPPÉ

Diabetics: double the amount of ice or ice water to dilute the concentration of sugar.
Hypertensives: double the amount of ice or ice water to dilute the concentration of sugar.
Kidney stones: strawberries not recommended (oxalate content).

Medical note: not recommended for people with gastritis due to strawberries acidity.

FROZEN LEMONADE

Medical note: as far as possible, drink it natural (without sugar or sweeteners).

GREEN TEA WITH LEMON

Cardiacs: do not consume strong tea because caffeine concentration may produce tachycardia.
Kidney stones: tea not recommended (oxalate content).

Medical note: due to the high concentrations of caffeine in green tea, patients suffering from gastritis are advised to replace it with peach tea.

GREEN TEA WITH MINT AND GINGER

Cardiacs: do not consume strong tea because caffeine concentration may produce tachycardia.
Kidney stones: tea not recommended (oxalate content).

Medical note: due to the high concentrations of caffeine in green tea, patients suffering from gastritis are advised to replace it with peach tea.

* Dialyze: To remove the salts or minerals found in some foods, after washing it is necessary to cook them in a medium-sized pot of boiling water (without salt) until tender. Remove pan from heat and drain the vegetables in a colander. In more severe medical cases, it is necessary to dialyze the vegetables two or more times, discarding the water used in each dialysis
see technique for dialyzing vegetables.

Note: the consumption of glucose and its relationship with hypertension is still debated. However, we take the freedom to suggest low sugar intake if you have other cardiovascular risk factors, like being a smoker, having hypertension, hyperlipidemia, obesity, etc.
http://circ.ahajournals.org/cgi/content/full/106/4/523

ADDITIONAL MEDICAL INFORMATION

Dietary guidance for prevention of kidney stones

To prevent kidney stones or its recurrence is important to supervise food intake. The proper diet will depend on the type of kidney stone that the patients produce. The most frequent kidney stones formed are those constituted by **sodium urate** and/or made up of **calcium oxalate**.

Urate (sodium urate) **kidney stones** are prevented by using the same type of diet used to prevent and/or treat gouty arthritis. This disease is related to the high uric acid total body content and uric acid blood levels. It is important to note that although high urate levels in urine propitiate the apparition of kidney stones, there are patients with similar readings that do not suffer from gout or kidney stones. The total amount of **sodium urate** in the urine is determined by measuring total urate in the urine collected for 24 hours.

Medical treatment with *allopurinol* is effective in gouty patients (or urate kidney stones patients) that have high levels of uric acid in blood (and/or high **urate** in urine). However, a low purine diet is required when this drug fails to reduce adequately the uric acid blood levels and/or the total urate level in the 24 hours urine collection. This contrasts with the treatment of gouty patients with high uric acid levels in blood but low urate levels in the 24 hours urine collection. In this last case, the medical treatment is with *probenecid*, and the installment of a low purine diet.

The diet for gout suffering patients (or patients with sodium urate kidney stones) limits foods having a high content of purines, which are the uric acid precursors. It should be mentioned that *allopurinol* is so effective in controlling uric acid in blood (and **sodium urate** in urine) that for the great majority of patients, to try to lower these levels only through diet is a practice of the past.

Alcoholic beverages are generally rich in calcium, oxalate, and guanosine (which is further metabolised to uric acid). To avoid triggering gout attacks, it is imperative for these patients **not to consume alcohol**.

Those foods that contain high amounts of purines are: asparagus, cauliflower, spinach, mushrooms, green peas, lentils, beans, oats, wheat germ, and, especially some meats such as viscera, sardines, herring, anchovies and oysters. Among foods that contain small amounts of purines are eggs, tofu and nonfat dairy products.

Kidney stones made up of **calcium oxalate** are associated with a high excretion of **oxalate** and/or **calcium**, or **both**, in the 24 hours collected urine. The medical treatment and/or the proper nutrition are determined depending on whether the excretion of oxalate or calcium or both are high in the urine.

Patients with calcium oxalate stones that have a high calcium excretion in the 24 hours collected urine, not necessarily have a high oxalate excretion, so that the restriction of oxalate in the diet is not essential in this last case.

If there is high **calcium** excretion in the urine, the treatment consists of a salt-restricted diet and sometimes enhanced with an alkaline food diet (vegetables) to reduce calcium excretion in the urine (however this is controversial as alkaline urine can promote calcium oxalate crystallization). Treatment with *hydrochlorothiazide* (a diuretic) is very effective in preventing this type of stones.

The restriction of dairy products containing high amounts of calcium is not necessarily associated with a decreased risk of producing these stones. The absorption of calcium from food depends on the consumption of fats and oxalates in the diet.

A relatively low fat diet is recommended too because the fat in diet captures intestinal calcium (saponification). This allows dietary oxalate to be absorbed and excreted in larger amounts in the urine, thus favoring the formation of calcium oxalate kidney stones.

The restriction of calcium and dairy products in patients with **calcium oxalate** stones is indicated for only those patients having high intestinal calcium absorption and/or a kidney inability to reabsorb calcium. The latter is rare and it is determined when a high calcium excretion in the 24 hours urine is found to persist in a patient placed on a low calcium diet (or while on treatment with calcium chelants).

These conditions are diagnosed only when medical treatment and/or a low calcium diet does not control the recurrence of stone formation. It is fundamental to point out that the decrease in calcium intake is not advisable for patients because this mineral is essential for bone structure preservation.

In case there is a high **oxalate** excretion in the 24 hours urine collection, it is necessary to limit the intake of foods that contain high amounts of oxalates. This diet is necessary only for patients with proven high **oxalate** excretion in the 24 hours collected urine. This diagnosis is necessary because many patients with **calcium** stones do not have high levels of **oxalates in** the 24 hours **urine** collection.

Vitamin C is an oxalate precursor and therefore it is not recommended to take vitamin C pills. There are also gastrointestinal conditions that favor oxalate absorption. These complex diseases are generally associated with intestinal malabsorption and frequently occur in patients with intestinal bypass and/or gastrointestinal inflammatory disease.

Additional advices:

- Water is the medium that dissolves toxins and minerals. This is a fundamental reason for keeping patients well hydrated (at least 8 glasses of water a day). This to prevent any type of kidney stones. Consuming lemonade is a healthy option.
- A regular intake of vitamin B6, citrates and magnesium prevents the formation of kidney stones.
- A high protein diet acidifies the urine and decreases the risk of calcium oxalate stones.
- The vegetarian diet and the use of sodium bicarbonate alkalinizes urine, reducing the formation risk of sodium urate stones.

DIFFERENT REACTIONS TO FOODS

There are two types of adverse reactions to food: **immunological reactions** and **intolerance to certain foods**.

Adverse immunologic reactions are due to the reactivity or sensitivity of the immune system to a specific allergen. The immune system defends the organism at a cellular level (or by antibodies) from inert substances or living elements that are recognized as foreign to the individual.

The response of this system is expressed through a cellular reaction or by means of antibodies that allow the elimination of the specific antigen through the inflammatory phenomenon.

The cellular response originates in the T lymphocyte, and the antibody response in the B lymphocytes. These lymphocytes are distributed throughout the body, circulating through the lymphatic system, blood and tissues. The presence of significant amounts of lymphocytes in the digestive system responds to the need for continued vigilance in that organ to prevent the entry of pathogens.

The immune system does not recognize foods as strange to the body because they are degraded by digestive enzymes to its primary components (sugars, amino acids and triglycerides). That is why an adverse immune response to food is regarded as an anomaly. In other words, this happens when the body does not recognize ingested substances as nutrients.

These responses are manifested through a variety of mechanisms that the organism has to control or deactivate such substances. One such mechanism triggers an inflammatory process that causes an illness or a pathological reaction that is harmful to the body, without the cause being well established.

Some theories have hypothesized that poor digestion of food produces partially digested molecules, that when subsequently absorbed, triggers an immune reaction against this antigen (in this case, a specific food).

Other theories are inclined to the loss of immunological tolerance caused by congenital defects, while some other researchers believe that these reactions are due to evolutionary changes in the interaction of a "new" food (transgenic) with the human being immune system.

There are two major groups of inflammatory responses to foods: the inflammatory immune response to **gluten** and the allergic type response.

The inflammatory adverse response to gluten produces intestinal celiac disease, dermatitis herpetiformis, etc. These chronic diseases are due to immune recognition of the gluten molecule.

Gluten is a mixture of diverse proteins such as gliadin and glutenin, present in wheat, barley, rye, triticale (hybrid of wheat and rye), kamut (wheat Poulard or Australian) spelt (cereal adapted to harsh climates, humid and cold) and possibly oats (by crossed contamination).

Patients with celiac disease develop a severe intestinal malabsorption problem with long-term symptoms such as diarrhea, weight loss, etc. This reaction is due to a cellular inflammatory response at the gut level, and the presence of antibodies to gluten, the antigen found in the cereals already mentioned.

For **celiac patients** the only effective treatment is changing their diet to a gluten-free diet for life, in order to allow regeneration of the intestinal villi. Thus, the use of rice, corn and other grains that do not contain gluten represent a nutritional alterative for treating this disease.

A different problem is food allergy. In this particular case, the patient develops an acute immediate reaction due to the presence of IgE antibodies directed to a specific component of food, causing high amounts of histamine secretion from the mast cells of the body.

Mast cells are reactive cells found in many organ tissues of the body. When activated they release a number of inflammatory substances. This allergic reaction can be severe or anaphylactic (with airway obstruction, hypotension and vasomotor collapse) or mild, such as serum sickness (with skin rash, itching or inflammation of mucous membranes).

Raw or cooked foods like eggs, corn, soy, certain vegetables, cereals, legumes, seafood, certain fruits, etc., can trigger food allergy. It is important not to confuse this reaction to the reaction to cereals in celiac disease.

This book does not attempt to be a comprehensive food allergy treatise. However, is noteworthy to mention that an allergic food reaction requires a careful epidemiologic, clinical and laboratorial approach. To have an accurate diagnosis, it is necessary to determine the ultimate cause of this reaction, as the culprit antigen can be cloaked in another processed food source.

An exhaustive medical study will allow the identification and elimination of the responsible food. However many months or years later it might be reintroduced and consumed regularly every 3 to 4 days. If the allergic reaction is severe or compromises the respiratory airway, it is essential to identify the responsible food and its reintroduction may even be contraindicated for life.

Intolerance to a food is not an immunological or allergic reaction, but rather it is a gastrointestinal or systemic reaction caused by a toxin or a derivative of a food eaten. The reaction occurs by enzyme deficiencies and/or chemical responses, as well as psychological associations to a particular food.

Lactose intolerance is a common disorder. This adverse reaction presents with pain, diarrhea and abdominal bloating. Treatment requires the abstinence of milk products or the intake of lactase-treated milk or lactose-free products, such as soybean milk/cheese, etc. This intolerance is caused by the deficiency of the digestive enzyme lactase, and as all enzymatic deficiencies, it is associated with the individual genetic constitution.

Other unusual conditions of food intolerance that require specialized attention is favism, a genetic disease that is triggered by consumption of certain beans, and intolerance to phenylalanine, an amino acid that causes PKU, English acronym for phenylketonuria, an inherited disease that prevents the body metabolism of the amino acid phenylalanine present in food.

GLOSSARY OF CULINARY TERMS

Dress
Add condiments to a salad; garnish.

Level
Even to the spoon or teaspoon edge levels.

Grained rice
In Peru, it means that when cooking rice the grains do not stick and can be easily separated using a fork.

Slice thinly
To cut flat pieces very fine or thin.

Julienne technique
Cut into very thin strips.

Crêpe
The French word *crêpe* comes from the Latin *crispus*, which means crisp. It is a European culinary contribution made mainly of wheat, used to form a round thin mass. Usually used as a basis together with savory or sweet ingredients. In some regions it is confused with the pancake.

Crispy or crunchy
A crust consistency preparation.

Drain
Remove all excess liquid.

Let cook
Cook without moving food until it is fully cooked.

Garlic clove
One of the several small bulb in the garlic head.

Done to a turn
Being at the moment or in the best way it can be.

Broccoli florets
It refers to the small broccoli bunches not including the stems.

Stuffing
In a piece of uncooked meat (or other food), add strips of bacon, truffles, ham, vegetables, etc., by using a mechadora or a knife to supply different flavors and fat inside during cooking.

Sprinkle
Spray liquid on a food or surface.

Wok
Cookware from China, similar to a lightweight, round and deep frying-pan.

Macerate (marinate)
To soak a food in a seasoned liquid (vinegar, wine, fruit juice, herbs, etc.) for a certain time in order to preserve, flavor or soften it.

Precook or partially cooked
Food still medium raw.

Folding movements
Gradually combine ingredients with a spatula, with up and down blending movements, so white eggs will not deflate.

Omelet
Omelet, in French omelette, is a recipe made up with beaten egg, cooked in a non-stick frying pan with butter or oil. In order to fry the omelet, pour the egg mixture into a pan with hot oil. The handle of the frying pan must be moved so that mixture fills the bottom. It is left to curdle and with a spatula gently off the edges, then incline the pan, fold over the omelet and serve immediately.

Lemon zest
Lemon zest is used to add more flavor to foods. Use a simple grater and proceed to scrape the skin of lemon before washing. Care must be taken not to include the pulp or white part, as it is bitter. You can save the zest chilled in an airtight container for up to two weeks.

Shredded chicken breast
Chicken breast cooked and separated into thin threads.

Pinch
Small amount.

Meringue
Beat until stiff involves shaking the egg whites, no yolks, until they are stiff and have a white foam consistency.

To "beat" vigorously stir the egg whites in a bowl with a whisk or electric wire, or with a fork. The movement must be circular and continue so whites will slowly obtain a consistency similar to fresh snow.

Eggs must be very fresh and a pinch of salt can help to reach the point of meringue faster and with more consistency.

Set aside
Separate to use later on.

Soufflé
Soufflé (*souffler* in French, which means 'blow' or 'inflate') is a recipe made with different ingredients and beaten whites until stiff. It is characterized by the volume that the preparation reaches when cooked in the oven. Serve immediately to conserve its size.

Made in the USA
Las Vegas, NV
03 November 2026

57424059R00145